Advance Praise for

The Complete Guide to Aut

Even a routine checkup can be a challenge for people with autism of any age. Building on her years of experience as a Certified Registered Nurse Anesthetist who was diagnosed with autism in mid-life, Anita Lesko provides an invaluable act of two-way translation with this book: translating the world of medicine for autistic people and their families, and translating autistic experience for her fellow health-care professionals. Loaded with practical tips and new ways of thinking about familiar situations, this book is a must-read for parents, teachers, therapists, autistic people, and anyone on the front lines of health care.

> — *Steve Silberman*, New York Times *bestselling author of*
> NeuroTribes: The Legacy of Autism and the Future of Neurodiversity

Anita Lesko has gifted the autism community with this important, groundbreaking work that will become the essential volume on health care issues and patient-centered care for autistic individuals. There is no one person who is more qualified to write this seminal work than Anita, who is a renowned autistic self-advocate and a nurse anesthetist with decades of experience in medical settings. Health care professionals, educators, parents and autistic individuals all need to have this book as a critical resource, and are so fortunate to have a compassionate professional with Anita's expertise sharing her personal experiences, professional knowledge and practical advice. Thanks to Anita, autistic children and adults, and their families will now be able to navigate the maze of health care services with greater knowledge and confidence.

> — *Barry M. Prizant, Ph.D., CCC-SLP*
> *Adjunct Professor at Brown University*
> *Director, Childhood Communication Services (Cranston, RI)*

A first of its kind, Anita Lesko employs a life time of hard-earned insights as a person with autism on providing medical care for individuals with autism from intake, through examination, to treatment. With nearly 3 decades as a nurse anesthesiologist, Ms. Lesko's detailed and step by step guide empowers doctors, nurses, others in allied fields, as well as parents and those on with autism to provide the best medical care possible. A must read for anyone who provides health care for individuals on the autism spectrum.

> — *Stephen M. Shore, EdD. Internationally renowned educator, author,*
> *consultant and presenter, person with autism*

Anita Lesko combines her professional expertise as a certified registered nurse anesthetist with her personal experience as an autistic adult to offer those on healthcare teams an inside glimpse of strategies and supports to improve healthcare for individuals on the autism spectrum. Readers will benefit from her insights and guiding questions that frame topics such as communication, adapting environments, and navigating the care pathway from admission to recovery for inpatient admissions. Anita's easy to read style and approach to the topic make this book accessible for all involved in healthcare!

> — *Teal Benevides, PhD, MS, OTR/L*
> *Associate Professor at Department of Occupational Therapy at*
> *Augusta University College of Allied Health Sciences*

Anita has identified a real need, and come up with real answers.

> — *John Donvan and Caren Zucker, authors of* In a Different Key: The Story
> of Autism, *the Pulitzer Prize finalist and* New York Times *bestseller. Caren*
> *and John work for* ABC World News *and are News and Documentary*
> *Emmy Award Winners.*

Foreword by Dr. Temple Grandin

Advice for Medical Professionals and People on the Spectrum

The Complete Guide *to* AUTISM & Healthcare

Anita Lesko, BSN, RN, MS, CRNA

The Complete Guide to Autism & Healthcare

All marketing and publishing rights guaranteed to and reserved by:

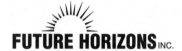

721 W. Abram Street
Arlington, TX 76013
(800) 489-0727
(817) 277-0727
(817) 277-2270 (fax)
E-mail: info@fhautism.com
www.fhautism.com

ISBN: 9781941765449

Dedication

I dedicate this book to my mom, Rita, and my husband, Abraham. Without Rita, I wouldn't have become the person I am today. Without Abraham, writing this book wouldn't have been possible. I dedicate this work also to my beloved cat, Callie Mae, affectionately called Baby Cakes, who spent many hours with me at the computer.

Contents

Foreword ix

Introduction xi

Chapter 1—What Is Autism? 1

Chapter 2—Demonstration Activity of Autism 11

Chapter 3—Looking through My Autistic Eyes at the Healthcare System 13

Chapter 4—Thinking Outside the Box 19

Chapter 5—Communicating with the Autistic Patient 21

Chapter 6—Sensory Issues and Sensory Processing Disorder 27

Chapter 7—Adaptation to the Environment 35

Chapter 8—Meltdowns & Safety 37

Chapter 9—Pain Perception of the Autistic Individual 43

Chapter 10—Preparing the Autistic Patient for an Exam or Procedure 47

Chapter 11—The Importance of Websites, Videos, and Albums 53

Chapter 12—Identification of Autistic Patients 59

Chapter 13—Emergency Department 61

Chapter 14—Inpatient Admissions 67

Chapter 15—Preparing for the Operating Room 79

Chapter 16—Anesthesia for the Autistic Patient 89

Chapter 17—Women's Health 101

Chapter 18—HIPAA Requirements 107

Chapter 19—Americans with Disabilities Act 109

Chapter 20—Putting All the Pieces Together 123

Chapter 21—Parents: The Unsung Heroes 129

Chapter 22—Conclusion 133

About the Author 135

Foreword

Anita Lesko is uniquely qualified to write about how health care professionals can make medical procedures more comfortable for children and adults on the autism spectrum. She has a successful career as a nurse anesthetist and, at age 50, she discovered that she was on the autism spectrum. Even though loud noise and sensory over-sensitivity bothered her, she excelled in her profession. Today, she administers anesthesia for complex brain operations and organ transplants, and is specializing in anesthesia for orthopedic joint replacement surgery. Attention to detail is required when working on such challenging cases.

The first rule in performing medical procedures on individuals with autism is: NEVER allow surprises. Surprises scare. Anita's book contains detailed instructions on how to explain medical procedures to a person with autism. Also, the person will be more relaxed if he or she can visit the facility before the procedure.

When I was a child, some medical procedures were done well and others resulted in a big meltdown. When I was about five years old, the doctor told me to look out the window at a bird feeder. He thought he could give me a shot and I would not notice it. When the needle went in, I screamed and had a tantrum. For future doctor's appointments, my mother developed a system. When we first arrived at the office, my doctor looked at my records to see if I needed any vaccinations. If the records showed that I needed no shots, I could relax because I knew no shots were coming. If I needed a shot, it was done first to get it over with, which made the rest of my medical exam peaceful.

At age six, I had to have my tonsils out. In the early 1950s, they still used ether and a mask that looked like a kitchen strainer. The room was quiet and the experienced nurse knew how to keep me calm. She momentarily put the mask to her face and showed that it did not hurt her, and then she gently put it on me. That is the last thing I remembered until I woke up with a very sore throat.

One of the most important things that medical professionals need to understand is the problems people with autism have with sensory over-sensitivity. Some individuals are disturbed by bright lights. Motion from a gurney being moved quickly may cause sensory overload. Other individuals cannot tolerate loud noise. Touch sensitivity is another problem area. Sensory over-sensitivity in autism is HIGHLY VARIABLE. One person with autism may have problems with visual over-sensitivity while another cannot tolerate loud sudden noises. If a person has touch-sensitivity problems, he or she may have trouble staying still when equipment touches the skin. At the eye doctor, I had to have a glaucoma test where a lens-like device was put against my eye. Staying still was almost impossible. I discovered a way to desensitize my eye. If I wore eye patches for fifteen minutes BEFORE the exam, putting in the lens was easy. The padded eye patches exerted slight pressure against my eyelids and desensitized them.

If a medical professional is working with fully verbal individuals who can easily communicate, I strongly recommend a discussion of the patient's SPECIFIC sensory problems. Each person is different and the sensory problems are extremely variable.

Dr. Temple Grandin, author

The Way I See It

The Autistic Brain

Introduction

The latest findings from the Centers for Disease Control in Atlanta show 1 in every 68 children are diagnosed as being on the autism spectrum. This translates into millions of individuals around the world with autism. This population has at least the same needs for health care as the general population, and even more so. Based on a study by epidemiologist Laura Schieve, Ph.D., of the National Center on Birth Defects and Developmental Disabilities, at the Centers for Disease Control and Prevention, it was concluded that children with autism have a much greater chance for respiratory issues, chronic gastrointestinal issues, allergies, and headaches.[1] Add anxiety to these ailments, and morbidity climbs even higher. Also, don't forget about autistic adults. The main focus has been on autistic children, but there are millions of adults on the autism spectrum, diagnosed or not; they might be your next patient!

Special strategies and accommodations are necessary to provide optimal care for autistic patients. Most importantly, healthcare professionals and all ancillary staff must understand autism. Only through understanding of autistic individuals can effective communication occur. The majority of autism focus is on children. Reality is that these autistic children will grow up to become autistic adults. Furthermore, there are millions of adults on the autism spectrum right now, many who avoid seeking medical attention. The reason they avoid health care is for lack of understanding from the health care providers, sensory overload, unwelcome touching, providers' assumptions about the patient, misunderstandings, and more. We need to change this.

From my own personal experiences and those of many others on the spectrum, it is quite evident there is a serious need for all healthcare professionals and ancillary staff to learn about autism. They must not only understand autism but also know how to communicate in various ways and optimize an environment to minimize sensory overload. Patients may be anywhere on the autism spectrum. There is no single way to communicate effectively with all individuals. Communication skills are typically among the most challenging to master for those with autism. In order to achieve optimal health care, health care providers must effectively communicate with each patient.

Additionally, communication must commence at the admissions desk and follow the patient through the final discharge. Whether simply coming for a routine doctor's appointment or getting admitted for major surgery, the autistic patient needs specialized care for optimal awareness, sensory processing, communication challenges, legal and ethical issues, compliance with HIPAA, compliance with the American's with Disabilities Act, and much more.

The book is designed for use by academic professionals in courses in the healthcare curriculum and as a guide for everyone working in the health care field. Below is a list of those who need to be well versed in autism.[2] By no means is this list complete; there are many more personnel who will benefit from this guide book.

Licensed Professionals:

- Speech Language Pathologists
- Occupational Therapists
- Physicians
- Dentists
- BCBA and ABA Professionals
- Physical Therapists

- Psychologists
- Clinical Social Workers
- Licensed Professional Counselors
- RN Nurses
- Recreational Therapists

Education Professionals:

- Special Education Teachers
- Special Education Directors
- School Psychologists
- Behavior Specialists

- School Counselors
- Classroom Teachers
- Principals

To all who shall read this book, I'd like to make a statement for you to always keep in your mind. I have the pleasure of knowing and calling as my friends Dr. Temple Grandin and her mother, Eustacia Cutler. Temple offered the toast at my all-autistic wedding, and Eustacia called in remotely during the cake-cutting ceremony with a special message. When Temple was a young child, Eustacia coined a phrase that Temple used for the title of a book. She stated that autistic individuals are "different, not less."

Introduction

Despite the (at times) bizarre differences between autistic and non-autistic people, we truly do have the same basic needs like love, relationships, acceptance, and happiness, just like everyone else. We experience the world very differently than others, thus the way we respond is just as different.

Footnotes

1. Schieve LA, Gonzales V, Boulet SL, Visser SN, Rice CE, Van Naarden-Braun K, Boyle CA. Concurrent medical conditions and health care use and needs among children with learning and behavioral developmental disabilities, *National Health Interview Survey*, 2006-2010. Res Dev Disabil. 2011;33:467-76.

2. List obtained from the International Board of Credentialing and Continuing Education Standards. www.ibcces.org

Chapter 1 ——————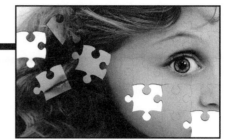
What Is Autism?

This chapter shall commence with a description of autism obtained by the most credible sources on earth. Following that will be a discussion of what it's like to live with autism and a first-hand account of how differently we perceive the world.

According to the Centers for Disease Control (CDC) in Atlanta, Autism spectrum disorder (ASD) is a developmental disability that can cause significant social, communication, and behavioral challenges. Often there is nothing about how a person with ASD looks that sets him or her apart from other people, but people with ASD may communicate, interact, behave, and learn in ways that are different from most other people. The learning, thinking, and problem-solving abilities of people with ASD can range from gifted to severely challenged. Some people with ASD need a lot of help in their daily lives; others need less.

A diagnosis of ASD now includes several conditions that used to be diagnosed separately: autistic disorder, pervasive developmental disorder not otherwise specified (PDD-NOS), and Asperger's syndrome. These conditions are now all included in the term autism spectrum disorder. [3]

The Autism Society of America goes into more detail on the definition of autism, as follows:

> Autism spectrum disorder (ASD) is a complex developmental disability; signs typically
> appear during early childhood and affect a person's ability to communicate and interact
> with others. ASD is defined by a certain set of behaviors and is a spectrum condition that
> affects individuals differently and to varying degrees. There is no known single cause of

autism, but increased awareness, early diagnosis/intervention, and access to appropriate services/supports lead to significantly improved outcomes. Some of the behaviors associated with autism include delayed language learning; difficulty making eye contact or holding a conversation; difficulty with executive functioning, which relates to reasoning and planning; narrow, intense interests; poor motor skills; and sensory sensitivities. Again, a person on the spectrum might follow many of these behaviors or just a few, or many others besides. The diagnosis of autism spectrum disorder is applied based on an analysis of all behaviors and their severity.[4]

Signs of autism will begin before a child reaches his third birthday and will remain with him throughout his entire life. Symptoms can lessen as the individual gets older, to the point that it's barely recognized as an adult. However, the person will still struggle with many of the issues as an adult, as they never go completely away. Many on the autism spectrum have extraordinary gifts beyond what ordinary people have that bring much happiness and fulfillment to them.

Some children might show signs or symptoms of autism within the first few months of life; while in others, symptoms might not surface until they are twenty-four months old. Some children might appear to develop normally until age two, then suddenly stop gaining new skills and lose the ones they have. There is no exact pattern and development, which is why it is called a spectrum.

The CDC has lists of signs and symptoms for various areas that are shown below.[5] It is not unusual for parents to see these lists and suddenly realize that their child fits the picture, or for an adult suddenly to realize she is on the spectrum, never understanding why she was so different.

Possible Red Flags

A person with ASD might:

- Not respond to her name by 12 months of age
- Not point at objects to show interest (point at an airplane flying over) by 14 months

- Not play "pretend" games (pretend to "feed" a doll) by 18 months

- Avoid eye contact and want to be alone

- Have trouble understanding other people's feelings or talking about her own feelings

- Have delayed speech and language skills

- Repeat words or phrases over and over (echolalia)

- Give unrelated answers to questions

- Get upset by minor changes

- Have obsessive interests

- Flap her hands, rock her body, or spin in circles

- Have unusual reactions to the way things sound, smell, taste, look, or feel

Social issues are one of the main challenges associated with ASD. These difficulties can cause serious problems in these people's everyday lives.

Examples of social issues related to ASD:[6]

- Does not respond to his name by 12 months of age

- Avoids eye contact

- Prefers to play alone

- Does not share interests with others

- Only interacts to achieve a desired goal

- Has flat or inappropriate facial expressions

- Does not understand personal space boundaries

- Avoids or resists physical contact

- Is not comforted by others during distress

- Has trouble understanding other people's feelings or talking about his own feelings

Every parent wants a perfect child. Parents typically spend time socializing with other parents of children the same age to exchange stories of their child's progress. I'm all too familiar with this event; it occurs regularly in my own workplace. As I listen to my colleagues sharing stories about their child's progress, I wonder to myself how each of them would act if their child was diagnosed with autism and was four years old and still not talking or reaching any of the "normal" development milestones. People take for granted that they will have a "normal" child.

By a child's first birthday, she is typically very interested in people and the world around her. An autistic child might not have any interest in others or the world around her. This is the beginning of a long journey of learning how to interact with people and navigate life in general.

Communication

One of the biggest difficulties someone with ASD will face is communication. Not only will an autistic individual have difficulties communicating, but he will also face difficulty in understanding others in both verbal and non-verbal forms of communication. For many, this will improve over time, but for many it will not.

Each person with ASD has different communication skills. Some people can speak well, while others can't speak at all or only very little. About 40% of children with an ASD do not talk at all. About 25% to 30% of children with ASD have some words at 12 to 18 months of age and then lose them. Others might speak, but not until later in childhood.[7]

Examples of communication issues related to ASD:[8]
- Demonstrates delayed speech and language skills
- Repeats words or phrases over and over (echolalia)
- Reverses pronouns (e.g., says "you" instead of "I")
- Gives unrelated answers to questions
- Does not point or respond to pointing
- Uses few or no gestures (e.g., does not wave goodbye)
- Talks in a flat, robot-like, or sing-song voice

- Does not pretend in play (e.g., does not pretend to "feed" a doll)

- Does not understand jokes, sarcasm, or teasing

The National Institute of Child Health and Human Development (NICHD) lists five behaviors that warrant further evaluation:

- Does not babble or coo by 12 months

- Does not gesture (point, wave, grasp) by 12 months

- Does not say single words by 16 months

- Does not say two-word phrases on his or her own by 24 months

- Has any loss of any language or social skill at any age

While any of these symptoms do not necessarily indicate a child has autism, occurrence of them warrants an evaluation by a multidisciplinary team. This team would include a neurologist, psychologist, developmental pediatrician, speech/language therapist, learning consultant, or other professional knowledgeable about autism.[9]

Unusual Interests and Behaviors

Many people with ASD demonstrate unusual interest or behaviors.

Examples of unusual interests and behaviors related to ASD:

- Lines up toys or other objects

- Plays with toys the same way every time

- Likes parts of objects (e.g., wheels)

- Is very organized

- Gets upset by minor changes

- Has obsessive interests

- Has to follow certain routines

- Flaps hands, rocks body, or spins self in circles

People with ASD typically thrive on routine. Any little change in their routine can greatly upset them to the point of having a meltdown. They can have unusual reactions to touch, sounds, smells, tastes, and textures. This is due to the fact that their sensory levels are extremely intense compared to others.

Another list from the CDC includes the following.[10]

Other Symptoms

Some people with ASD have other symptoms. These might include:

- Hyperactivity (very active)
- Impulsivity (acting without thinking)
- Short attention span
- Aggression
- Causing self-injury
- Temper tantrums
- Unusual eating and sleeping habits
- Unusual mood or emotional reactions
- Lack of fear or more fear than expected
- Unusual reactions to the way things sound, smell, taste, look, or feel

Children with ASD develop at different rates and in different areas. It is not unusual for an autistic child to progress very rapidly in one particular area, such as mathematics, yet be far behind in simple areas. A child might become a computer whiz yet be unable to socialize with other children her own age.

Adults with ASD may function at various ranges on the spectrum. Many adults over 30 are diagnosed late in life. This is due to the fact that much knowledge on the subject was not translated into the United States until 1994. Until that point, those who are now adults had gone under the radar, either getting incorrect diagnoses or no diagnosis at all.

Chapter 1: What Is Autism?

I personally did not get diagnosed until the age of fifty, and that was only by accident. A co-worker's son had just been diagnosed with Asperger's Syndrome. When she handed me a few papers with information about Asperger's, the top sheet showed a list stating that if you have ten out of twelve of the symptoms listed, you have Asperger's. I had twelve out of twelve. That night I stopped off at the local book store and purchased every book on the shelf about Asperger's Syndrome. Once I got home, the first one that caught my eye was by Dr. Tony Attwood, *The Complete Guide to Asperger's Syndrome*.

I stayed up all night reading it, crying most of the way, and by the dawn's early light I knew without a doubt that I had Asperger's. Three weeks later, I had my formal diagnosis from a neuropsychologist. That testing occurred over a three-day period with a series of psychological tests which took about 3 to 4 hours on each of those days, followed by a very lengthy visit with the neuropsychologist.

Until now, the main focus of most literature has been on autistic children. Finally, people are recognizing there are autistic adults, literally millions of them, and millions more will come as today's autistic children grow up to become adults.

Sadly, it is not uncommon for autistic adults to avoid going for routine health care due to the sensory issues involved, unwanted touching, and lack of understanding by healthcare providers. What typically happens is that these adults neglect a problem until it reaches a level of emergency. By that point, not only is the issue at a critical point, but it is also compounded by the massive sensory overload of the emergency room, and an emotional meltdown may occur. After sitting in a loud, brightly lit waiting area, with TVs typically going, multiple other people sitting in close proximity, the smells of cleaning fluids and disinfectants, and phones endlessly ringing, the autistic individual will be at his wits' end by the time his name is called to be taken into an exam room. Once in a room waiting to be seen by a nurse or physician, the person might be at a point of breakdown. This could seriously affect the way he processes whatever information is provided for the direction of his treatment and follow-up care. By taking simple measures, the environment in healthcare facilities can be changed to accommodate autistic patients. Even small changes can go a long way. These changes will be discussed at length later in the book.

Autism occurs in every race and at every socioeconomic level. It has no borders, and is found in every country around the globe. Boys are diagnosed more often than females. While the individual will never be "cured" of autism, it generally gets better over time. In today's world, it is typical that, once a child gets diagnosed with autism, intervention immediately begins. Early intervention is the key to enabling the individual to become the most that he can be. Some people, like me, never had any kind of intervention. What I did have, however, was a mother who devoted her entire life to me, and her unwavering support enabled me to achieve all that I have accomplished in my lifetime thus far. This factor will also be discussed later in the book.

Despite our different ways, always remember that we are different, but not less. Embrace your autistic patients, for so many of us have gifts to enrich this world. We also want to be loved, to love, and have relationships, just like everyone else.

Having gone the first fifty years of my life undiagnosed puts me in a very different category from the young people of today who get diagnosed in early childhood. Aside from the fact that I didn't receive any kind of intervention, I spent all those years wondering why I was so different, why I never fit in, why I was unable to make or keep any friends, and why I had a myriad of sensory issues that no one else seemed to have. I always felt like I was on the outside of life, looking in at everyone else, wondering why I couldn't be like them.

After getting diagnosed, my whole life changed in a very positive way. I was greatly relieved to finally understand why I was like this and that I wasn't alone any longer. A common theme to autistic individuals is loneliness. Despite the challenges I faced all throughout my life, I would not want to have known sooner about my autism. I see so many autistic individuals who do get diagnosed early in life, and that then becomes their focus in a very negative way. At this point in my life, my goal is to change the world's view of autism. I also want to help healthcare providers understand autism and to show them ways they can improve autistic patients' experiences in obtaining their health care. That will enable the autistic population to readily seek not only urgent care, but also to feel comfortable going for routine health screenings and maintenance.

Footnotes

3. Centers for Disease Control, Atlanta https://www.cdc.gov/ncbddd/autism/facts.html

4. Autism Society of America http://www.autism-society.org/what-is/

5. Centers for Disease Control, Atlanta, https://www.cdc.gov/ncbddd/autism/facts.html

6. CDC (https://www.cdc.gov/ncbddd/autism/signs.html)

7. CDC (https://www.cdc.gov/ncbddd/autism/signs.html)

8. CDC- https://www.cdc.gov/ncbddd/autism/signs.html

9. http://www.autism-society.org/what-is/symptoms/

10. https://www.cdc.gov/ncbddd/autism/signs.html

Chapter 2 Demonstration

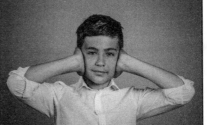

Activity of Autism

I am very lucky to have had Dr. Stephen Shore as a close friend. He is best known as the Globetrotting Autism Ambassador! He had been diagnosed at age two with autism, and it was suggested to his parents that they should consider institutionalization as the best place for him. Thankfully, his parents didn't listen to those professionals. Early intervention was immediately started upon Stephen's diagnosis, much by his own family.

Stephen earned a PhD and is a professor at Adelphi University for Special Education. He also focuses on research for matching best practice to the needs of people with autism. In addition to working with autistic children and talking about life on the autism spectrum, Stephen is internationally renowned for his presentations, consultations, and writings on lifespan issues pertinent to education, relationships, employment, advocacy, and disclosure.[11]

I feel that, in order for the reader of this book to best understand autism, participating in a simulation is an excellent way to get a better understanding of how we perceive the world and the massive sensory overload that goes with autism. What we experience is far beyond the activity shown below, but by engaging in this exercise, you will at least gain some understanding (and compassion, I hope!) of this very different way of life. You will need each group to have five people.

Stephen M. Shore, Ed.D.   **Autism Spectrum**   sshore@adelphi.edu

S E N S O R Y   O V E R L O A D   A C T I V I T Y

In groups of 5, each person plays a specific role. Start when given the signal

Person #1: You play the role of a person with autism. Your job is to listen to what Person #5 is reading to you so you can take a test on the material. Try to ignore everyone else.

Person #2: Stand behind the student playing the part of someone with autism. Rub the edge of an index card (or piece of cardboard) against the back of their neck. You do not need to rub hard, but keep doing it over and over.

Person #3: Grab a book (any book will do), lean close to Person #1 and read in a loud voice the entire time.

Person #4: Pat Person #1 on the head and shoulder the entire time.

Person #5: Using a normal voice, read a paragraph to Person #1 then ask them questions about what you read. Do NOT try to drown out the other noises.

Have all the group members take a turn being Person #1.
- How did it feel to have so much commotion going on?
- Did it make you want to scream and run away?
- Was Person #1 able to concentrate on the paragraph being read?
- What might have helped?

Adcock, B., & Remus, M. (2006). *Disabilities awareness activity packet: Activities and resources for teaching students about disabilities.* Possibilities, inc, p. 4. Available on February 19, 2011 at http://www.vcu.edu/partnership/C-SAL/downloadables/PDF/DisabilityAwarenessPacket.pdf.

Once you have completed the Sensory Overload activity, you will probably have a very different perspective of your next autistic patient! Most people who participate in the activity want to simply get away from all the stimuli. Lucky for you, you can simply run away from it! An autistic person can't run away from it, and it's a way of life for us 24/7, 365 days a year. I often describe it as living in Dolby surround sound. Have you ever walked into a store that sells TVs, and they have like fifty TVs all playing at the same time? That's the magnitude of sensory input we experience daily.

Footnotes

11. www.autismasperger.net/bio.htm

Chapter 3

Looking through My Autistic Eyes at the Healthcare System

Just prior to graduating from college with my Bachelor of Science in Nursing in 1983, I broke my arm while ice skating. For a number of years, I'd been into ice dancing, and on a cold December day, I had an accident while practicing some new moves on the ice. I heard a loud snap as my left arm hit the ice first. As I got up, I could see there was a fracture, as the arm was now crooked. Little did I know at the time that the incident would change my life in a very big way.

Once at the local hospital in the Emergency Department, I sat awaiting an orthopaedic surgeon who was coming in to reduce the fracture and apply a cast on my arm. An anesthesiologist arrived, and he began assembling some syringes and medications for my sedation. He asked what I do, to which I replied that I was earning my BSN. He then suggested I go to be a nurse anesthetist. I'd never heard of this, so he explained what it was. Hearing that I could earn a Master's degree and learn how to give anesthesia for all types of surgery and even do spinal taps, epidurals, and invasive monitoring piqued my interest.

In 1988, I graduated from Columbia University in New York City with my Master of Science in Nurse Anesthesia. As I write, I'm going into my 28th year working full time as a Certified Registered Nurse Anestheist (CRNA). Of all those years, the first 22 were quite the struggle regarding social interactions. I didn't yet know about my autism at that time. But when I discovered I'm autistic, my view of the healthcare system didn't change. Not one bit.

I'm going to discuss this point from two points of view: first will be my perception as a CRNA, and the other will be as a patient.

My career as a CRNA has actually been my therapy in a way. It forced me to interact with people, hundreds of thousands of people, and in fact, I've recently calculated it to be over one million interactions with people. For any "normal" person with a job that entails interacting with endless people, that isn't so impressive. For an individual with autism, however, I'm in a class all by myself.

In chapter one I discussed the fact that, as an autistic individual gets older, his symptoms generally get better, including the ability to communicate with others. This was certainly true in my case. Looking back, I cringe as I remember my younger days and my autistic ways! I can well remember saying things that I know would sent people into a tailspin. I simply didn't know how to interact with people; I was always saying the wrong thing, or the right thing in the wrong tone! I couldn't understand why people would be so upset at me for something I'd say. I was clueless.

I have been a people watcher my whole life. I'd study the behaviour of others, but never understand why I was so different from them. Shopping malls on a busy Saturday would make an excellent place to get a coffee and watch the crowd. It was fascinating to observe every facial expression, every conversation and every move people made. The most frustrating thing was that it was all foreign to me. Nothing of what I was watching was even close to anything I did. Why, I wondered, was I so different? That feeling always crept in, that I was on the outside of life looking in. Oh, I wanted to get in, but I simply couldn't find the door to walk into that other world.

The side I was on was lonely, and I'd try to make friends. On the rare occasion that I did make a friend, it was very short lived. I can remember once watching the *Oprah Winfrey Show*, and Oprah had on her best friend, Gayle King. She was talking about how wonderful it was having Gayle as her best friend for the past twenty years.

Chapter 3: Looking through My Autistic Eyes at the Healthcare System

I burst out crying, as I'd never had a best friend, not ever. I felt even more odd and lonely than ever before. I often felt like I was from some other planet, an alien to this one.

All of this changed the day I learned about Asperger's and that I was on the spectrum. But some things really didn't change, including my perception of the healthcare system!

As a nurse anesthetist, I've seen many things over the past twenty-eight years. My sensory issues have been the biggest obstacle throughout my career, and still affect me to this day. When I think about it, working in the operating room environment is probably the worst career choice for someone on the spectrum due to the massive sensory overload there.

There are bright surgical lights directly over the operating table so the surgeons can see well. An anesthesia provider stands directly at the head of the table, and these bright lights shine my way. That's a sensory violation, as my friend Stephen Shore calls it! Surgeons frequently like to play heavy metal, or angry music, in the O.R., very loudly. I mean they play it so loud that I can't hear the monitors or the O.R. staff talking in the room. I try very hard to cope with the loud music, but after a short time I simply can't.

My brain functions like a computer. At any given time, I "see" six computer screens running. If one more screen "opens up," then they'll all crash, just like a search engine getting overloaded! The same holds true in the OR. I've got to focus on the patient, the monitors, IV fluids, ventilator, surgeons, and OR staff. I can easily keep track of all of these at the same time on my six "screens." But then add heavy metal blasting loud, and it sends me over the edge. Here's what happens: I'll get a massive, raging headache, which makes me feel sick all over. I'm still able to focus on my job, only now I'm physically suffering. I will politely ask if the volume can be turned down. Sometimes I'm accommodated, other times I get cursed out by the surgeon who makes some statement like, "I don't care about your f—king Asperger's" or some such thing. I finally got my department to simply not assign me to the rooms where that kind of music will be played.

Smells. There are numerous cases that involve smells I simply can't handle. One example, for starters, is the bovie, the cauterizing device, which produces electrosurgical smoke. Aside from the fact that this smoke is carcinogenic, it smells horrible. I'll watch in astonishment as others in the room are breathing this in with no hint of distaste for it, while I'm there with a double mask on, gagging at the plumes of smoke billowing up as the surgeon cauterizes the flesh. Of course there are cases involving smells from things like necrotizing fasciitis, or gangrene. That makes even the OR staff gag, so you can imagine what I'm like in a case like that. You get the picture!

Sounds—besides the heavy metal music, there are many sounds that occur in an operating room. Bone saws are one of them. I'm currently doing mostly orthopedics for joint replacements. Those doctors use bone saws, hammers, and all kinds of heavy instruments that make a lot of noise. I can remember a funny incident during which Stephen Shore happened to call me while I was in the OR doing a hip revision case. The surgeon started sawing bone. Stephen immediately asked what that horrific sound was. As I replied it was the bone saw, he stated that he couldn't take it, and he hung up. I thought it was pretty funny, as not only was I hearing the bone saw, but the bright surgical lights were shining at me, there was hard rock playing loudly, six people were all talking, all the sounds from the monitors (EKG, pulse oximeter, etc.) surrounded me, and I had occasional plumes of bovie smoke. Every possible sensory violation was happening. But this is just my daily life. Somehow, over the years, I've developed a tolerance for all of those factors. I would call it being desensitized, much like the process used to train police horses.

From an autistic patient point of view, just the thought of making a doctor's appointment makes me cringe. In my mind, I instantly conjure up numerous images. Because I think in pictures or in movie-like imagery, I instantly envision the whole gamut of what will happen. First, I'll arrive at the office and sign in at the window. I'll cringe at the sight of nearly every seat filled in the waiting room. If I can't find a seat where I'm by myself, I'll stand against the wall so I don't have to sit next to anyone. There will typically be a TV on to entertain the crowd there, because they're in for a long haul of waiting. Typically, there will be a news channel playing, with some unpleasant ads that surely will come on, in twice the volume of the news program. Some of those ads are extremely embarrassing to hear while in mixed company. But there you sit, or stand, with nowhere to hide, for a minimum of an hour, sometimes longer.

I laugh at all the HIPAA regulations that are supposed to protect a patient's privacy. There you are, sitting in a waiting room full of fifty other people, and a nurse steps out of the doorway and literally yells your name out, loud and clear. That HIPAA stuff just went flying out the window, as now everyone in that room just heard your name. Why is it that some eating establishments give you a buzzer when your order is ready, yet healthcare facilities yell your name out? Why isn't each patient issued a buzzer, so when it's your time to be taken into the exam room, your buzzer goes off? Then your patient privacy would actually be observed and respected.

While sitting (or standing) in the waiting area, there's bright lights, lots of people, and all kinds of smells from perfumes, colognes, body odor, and the frustration of excessive time in this myriad of sensory violations. Finally, after your name is yelled out, and everyone looks at you, you follow the nurse into an austere exam room. That will be your next place to wait yet again, occasionally up to an hour or longer. Typically, a nurse takes your blood pressure, temperature, and pulse, often in total silence, which makes me even more uncomfortable. I will always ask what my blood pressure is; otherwise she keeps it a secret as she logs it into the computer, then walks out the door. At least in this setting there are no people or TVs, just silence. But there might be smells from disinfectants or cleaning solutions of some sort. The longer I sit there, the more my anxiety grows. Suddenly there is a knock on the door, as it then slowly opens. In walks the doctor. Out reaches his hand to shake mine, with all the bacteria on his hand from the previous thirty patients he's just seen. I am a germ freak, and on rare occasions I've asked the doctor to wash his hands or at least use some hand disinfectant gel, both of which are readily available right there in the exam room. Each time I've requested that, I get a very negative response, where the doctor makes it very obvious that he is highly offended that I ask such a thing. That in turn makes me offended, as it is my right to be protected from other patients, and the standards come from JCAHO (Joint Commission on Accreditation of Healthcare Organizations) regulations to wash your hands prior to touching each patient. At this point, after waiting in excess of an hour and a half, my sensory overload is maxed out, and now the infested handshake. I'm not in a very pleasant mood at this point.

Then comes the touching. Autistic individuals generally don't like to be touched, especially by strangers, including healthcare professionals. I can't stand even when the nurse takes my blood pressure and must touch me. Then comes the stethoscope, which is put all over my chest and back, followed by whatever other touching the nurses must do. I dread it, and I cringe inside at each touch.

Fortunately, I am an excellent communicator at this point in my life. I can convey very easily to the doctor why I'm there, what's bothering me, where pain is at, and what type of pain it is. Other autistic individuals are not that proficient at communication, and that can be extremely detrimental to the interaction between the autistic patient and healthcare provider. By the time the patient has sat in the sensory overloaded waiting area and then the exam room, he is most likely on the verge of a meltdown. Compound this with not being able to communicate well, and a negative outcome is sure to follow. Additionally, then the autistic patient starts getting touched by the healthcare provider, generally without warning, and now you have a very unhappy patient.

As a healthcare provider myself, I know what's going to happen next while waiting at a doctor's office, getting blood drawn, getting an MRI, or even going for surgery. Even with that knowledge, I dread it all and will put off going for anything. Other autistic individuals who aren't healthcare providers won't know what's coming next, and everything will be extremely anxiety producing. Because of this, it is not uncommon for autistic adults to neglect their health.

My goal is to change all of this. In January 2016, I founded the Global Autism Consulting Organization with this Mission Statement:

"To Improve the Health and Wellbeing of Autistic People Around the World." — Anita Lesko

This book is part of my journey to reach my goal. I truly hope you will follow me on this mission.

We cannot have a population of people who are unhealthy just because they feared going for health care. As a fellow healthcare provider, and an autistic one, I ask you to always remember that we are "different, not less."

Chapter 4
Thinking Outside the Box

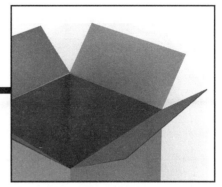

As a healthcare provider, I know from all my twenty-eight years in the profession that we folk always think that we know everything and what's best for a patient. That generally holds true in most cases, except for in the case of autistic patients, mainly autistic children. You will never find a parent more connected to their child than a parent of an autistic child. From the moment the child gets diagnosed with autism, the parent, typically the mother, becomes obsessed with that child. The early interventions begin as does the never-ending chain of therapy, counseling, IEP's, etc. These parents spend all their time with the child, Google every aspect of autism, join autism support groups for parents, and seek out any avenue of support or guidance they can find. They know every last detail of that autistic child. No one knows it better than that parent.

You need to truly LISTEN TO THE PARENTS!!! I can't stress this enough. They will be your biggest source of information for their autistic child (who might be a 45-year-old man!). I also highly suggest that you include the parents in the planning of care for the patient. Make them feel included in this aspect, and that effort will go a long way in long-term compliance.

I realize this isn't the norm for all of the patients that will cross your path. It is a new way of approaching patient care. This process might come as a struggle to some, but hopefully once you see the intensive involvement of the parent in that autistic child's life, you'll welcome their input and happily get her involved. By so doing, you will also gain that parent's trust.

On another note, it has been proven that many healthcare providers delayed autism diagnosis by ignoring parent concerns. A study done in 2011 clearly shows that many healthcare providers dismiss parents' early concerns about autism. Unfortunately, this resulted in significant delays in autism diagnosis and treatment. The parents initially begin raising concerns about possible autism symptoms when their child is around 2 years old. Sadly, these children weren't being diagnosed until close to 5 years of age. A lot of time was obviously lost through this occurrence.[12]

If a parent brings his child in and tells you he believes the child may be autistic, it's best to follow up on that feeling and proceed with getting the child evaluated. That parent is with the child 24/7 and knows exactly what signs and symptoms she is displaying. What you see during an office visit will not be representative of what the child is doing at home. It's better to be safe than sorry. The CDC has an excellent website entitled Learn the Signs. Act Early.[13]

Developmental Pediatrician Dr. Paul Wang, Autism Speaks' head of medical research, states, "we know that the earlier intervention gets started, the better the long-term outcome. Autism can get diagnosed as early as 18 months.[14]

In conclusion, be prepared to think outside the box!

Footnotes

12. www.cdc.gov/nchs/slaits/spds.htm

13. www.cdc.gov/ncbddd/actearly/index.html

14. www.autismspeaks.org/science/science-news/many-doctors-have-delayed-autism-diagnosis-ignoring-parent-concerns

Chapter 5

Communicating
with the Autistic Patient

Autism Spectrum Disorder (ASD) is so named for a very good reason. There are individuals at one end of the spectrum who cannot speak or need total assistance with activities of daily living, and at the other end of the spectrum are highly gifted people who are brilliant and need no assistance at all. There is a wide range of symptoms, severity, skills, and level of disability.

The word "autism" has its origin in the Greek word *autos*, which means *self*. Children with ASD tend to seem as if they exist in a private world, self-absorbed, unable to successfully communicate with others or interact with them. Children with ASD may have difficulty developing language skills and understanding what others say to them. Additionally, they might also have difficulty with nonverbal communication, such as eye contact, facial expressions, and hand gestures.[15]

It can be quite challenging for healthcare providers to consider the vast differences between individuals with ASD. Not every child will have difficulties with communication. Some have no ability to speak, while others have extreme ability to talk about their favorite interests in great detail. Those who can talk typically have difficulty using language effectively when talking to others. They may also have difficulty processing what they hear, and not understand what was said to them. For example, if an autistic child or adult is given verbal instructions on how to complete a task, she might not understand how to do it. Yet, if she is given an actual demonstration for the same task, she is then able to successfully do it herself. It's not uncommon for parents to think their child has hearing issues, because she doesn't respond when spoken to. The parents then take the child for hearing testing, only to learn there is no hearing deficit.

People with ASD are also unable to understand body language or the nuances of vocal tones. Body language is the second form of communication that humans use to express their thoughts, emotions, and desires. Those with ASD typically have difficulty at best, but usually no skills at deciphering what a person is saying with facial expressions or body language. A person with ASD also struggles to make eye contact. Many in fact will describe trying to look someone in the eye as being actually painful.[16]

Now that you have an overview of the communication difficulties of those with ASD, you are probably wondering exactly how you can effectively interact with your next autistic patient, wherever they may be on the autism spectrum. The ASD patient may appear not to hear what you say to him, he may not respond to his name, or he may appear indifferent to any attempts you make at communicating with him.

Tips for Communicating with the Autistic Patient

The first thing you need to do is take the ASD patient and her parents/support person to a very quiet, private room that is dimly lit, with minimal medical equipment in the room. There shouldn't be other patients or staff in the room. You want to create a relaxed, peaceful environment. That will calm the individual down. You will decrease the amount of sensory overload that affects the patient. I will go into a very detailed discussion about sensory issues in Chapter 6.

The next thing you need to do is ask the parent how the child/adult typically communicates. Parents can provide a baseline expectation of how the patient will react to you. Observe the way the patient communicates with her parent or whomever she is with. You will observe if she uses words or any type of gestures. Ask the parents for suggestions on how you should approach the patient. This goes back to Chapter 4 ("Thinking Outside the Box!"). Remember, that parent is with that child 24/7 and knows her every move. They are your best resource for your patient. You can also use this time to get the patient's medical history. Additionally, by allowing the patient to observe you talking to her parent, you will be establishing trust with her.

Say Less and Say It Slowly, but Not Too Slowly!

- Limit the amount of words you use to communicate with the ASD patient.

- Use key words that are specific to the situation. You may need to repeat and emphasize them, and accompany your words with simple gestures such as pointing.

- If the patient has only recently begun to use words, you might only be able to use single words. Be sure you have the child's attention, or words will have no meaning.

- You might need to pause between words or short sentences to allow the patient time to process what you are saying. Being out of his routine and in an intimidating setting, he might need more time to get his words out. Be patient and allow him time to put his thoughts into words. Your flexibility can reduce his anxiety and make the situation a whole lot better!

- If possible, use simple gestures and visual supports; visual supports include pictures showing a procedure like taking blood pressure, or a doctor listening to a patient's lungs with a stethoscope. This will be discussed later in Chapter 13.[17]

- Presume competence. Approach the situation as if the patient can understand you. That is simply showing respect towards the individual. I have personally heard many autistic individuals express distaste towards healthcare providers who start out talking to them as if they are severely mentally challenged.

- Be careful not to use figurative language—Sarcasm, idiomatic expressions, or read-between-the-lines talk won't work. ASD people take things very literally.

How an ASD person communicates depends on what she is hearing. Dr. Temple Grandin describes her hearing like having a sound amplifier set on maximum loudness. Her ears are like a microphone that picks up every little sound. She describes being unable to talk on a phone when in a crowded place such as an airport. If she tries to tune out all the background noise, she also tunes out the person on the phone.[18]

Written Communication

Another point to be made is that an ASD patient might wish to use written communication as a means of interacting with the healthcare team. Some individuals will feel more comfortable using either hand-written notes or a keyboard of some type to communicate his needs to you. In any case, remain flexible and show your willingness to provide accommodations to the patient. And again, incorporate the parent or support person in the patient's care.[19] By doing so, you will go a long way in the patient's trust of you. Showing your knowledge of autism will result in a very positive experience for the ASD patient, and for you as well! Written communication may be conducted in the form of writing on a piece of paper or pad or texting from a phone, an iPad or similar device, or a laptop computer. Whichever one he chooses, simply go with the flow, allow him time, and be patient. Keep in mind that the person probably feels anxious and self-conscious and may be having great difficulty processing everything that's going on.

Another factor to aim for is to limit the number of healthcare workers caring for the ASD patient. Introducing new staff to the patient will add significant stress to them, so try and keep the number of staff in the room to a minimum.[20]

Provide Simple and Straight-to-the-Point Instructions

ASD patients often misunderstand complex instructions. They typically cannot read between the lines. They will take everything literally. Say exactly what you mean. If you are trying to hurry the ASD patient by saying "Step on it!", don't be surprised if they ask you what you want them to step on.[21]

Simplify your sentences and be straight to the point. If she asks questions, keep your answers direct to the point as well.[22]

A Word on Dysgraphia

Some children with ASD also have dysgraphia, or written expression disorder. This learning disability impacts a child's ability to write and spell without affecting her reading ability. Many people with dysgraphia have higher-than-average IQs. In young children, this disability can show up when learning how to write. In older children, it may surface in the form of having a hard time putting their thoughts on paper, even though they are orally able to explain their thoughts.[23]

Footnotes

15. www.nidcd.nih.gov/health/autism-spectrum-disorder-communication-problems-children

16. www.disabled-world.com/artman/publish/autism-language.shtml

17. www.autism.org.uk/about/communication/communicating.aspx

18. My Experiences with Visual Thinking Sensory Problems and Communication Difficulties. Dr. Temple Grandin

19. "Respect the way I need to communicate with you": Healthcare experiences of adults on the autism spectrum. Autism October 2015 19:824-831.

20. www.nursebuff.com/2015/12/nursing-care-for-autism

21. www.stanfordchildrens.org

22. www.nursebuff.com/2015/12/nursing-and-autism

23. www.healthcentral.com/autism/c/1443/146027/dysgraphia-disorder/

Chapter 6
Sensory Issues
and Sensory Processing
Disorder

I
f you have participated in the Sensory Overload Activity in Chapter 2, you have a basic understanding of what it's like to be autistic. I often describe it as living with Dolby surround sound going 24/7. You can never tune anything out. It is simply massive stimuli coming at you non-stop.

Recently I was in the pre-op area at 6:30am reviewing the chart of my first patient of the day. The room was going in full swing. Twenty patients were in their cubicles with family members in attendance, nurses scurrying about, surgeons coming in to see their patients and mark the surgical sites, phones ringing, pagers going off, dozens of simultaneous conversations, portable x-rays being done, people moving all over … a typical day in the operating room suite! I stopped for a moment and just stood there by the desk area and looked around at everything going on. My computer brain was beginning to get maxed out. As I looked on, several of the pre-op nurses were sitting right in front of me, tending to their paperwork. It was obvious to me that they were totally oblivious to all the activity and noise going on around them. I was reaching near melt-down stage. I decided to ask them how they can tolerate it all so well. When I presented them with my question, they looked at me quite puzzled. One of them responded, "What noise are you talking about?" I then looked at her in disbelief! Motioning with my head at all the patients, staff and noise, the nurse looked at me and said, "I just tune it all out. I wasn't aware of it until now that you've brought my attention to it all. Just tune it all out!" I stared at her and replied, "I can't just tune it all out!" She then stated, "Sure you can! You just tune it out!" By this point she was furrowing her brows at me. I recognized that as she was baffled as to why couldn't I simply just tune it all out. "Well," I started … "You don't have autism!" To which she said, "What's the big deal?" It makes all the difference in the world. Our brains just cannot flip a switch to stop our senses from taking in everything in an extremely magnified way.

Sensory Differences

Many people on the autism spectrum have difficulty processing everyday sensory information. Any of the senses may be over- or under-sensitive, or both, at different times. These sensory differences can affect behavior and can have a profound effect on a person's life.[24] Sensory processing disorder (SPD) is a condition that includes people who are overly sensitive to what they feel, see, and hear, but also those who are under sensitive, and still others who have trouble integrating information from multiple senses at once. SPD is not an official diagnosis. It isn't included in the newest edition of the "Diagnostic and Statistical Manual of Mental Disorders (DSM-5). Still, it is widely used as a catch-all by clinicians, and some studies suggest that it may affect between 5 and 15 percent of school-aged children.[24-a] To add further interest, a person with SPD is not necessarily autistic. However, a person with ASD will most likely have SPD.

Many of the day-to-day struggles of people with autism have to do with perceptions gone haywire, such as being overwhelmed by sounds, feeling a revulsion towards certain foods, or experiencing sensory overload from being touched. All of this has a major impact on the ASD individual's life.

Researchers are applying neurobiology findings to treatment studies of sensory processing disorder, such as Dr. Elysa Marco, director of sensory neurodevelopment and autism.

Sensory Integration—A Very Complex Issue for Those on the Autism Spectrum

Children and adults on the AS may have a dysfunctional sensory system. One or more sensory systems can either over or under react to stimulation. Although receptors for the senses are located in the peripheral nervous system (which includes everything except the brain and spinal cord), it is believed that the actual problem arises from neurological dysfunction in the central nervous system—the brain.

The integration and interpretation of sensory stimulation from the environment by the brain is an innate neurobiological process known as sensory integration. In contrast, when sensory input is not integrated or organized appropriately in the brain, varying degrees of problems may result. This would include problems in development, information processing, or behaviour. This is referred to as sensory integrative dysfunction.

Humans can experience, interpret, and respond to all the stimuli in our environment through the complex inter-relationship of the three basic senses: tactile, vestibular, and proprioceptive. They are also interconnected with vision and auditory system. These senses are critical to our survival.

Tactile System

The tactile system includes all the nerves under the skin's surface that send information to the brain. This includes temperature, pressure, light touch, and pain. These all function to perceive the environment and also as protective reactions for survival.

For those on the AS, it is quite common to display a dysfunction in the tactile system. This would include withdrawing from being touched, refusing to wear certain types of fabrics that have a rough texture, refusing to eat certain foods due to the texture, or disliking the feeling of running water on the body. A person with a dysfunctional tactile system will experience her environment (touch, pain, food, clothing) far differently from others. This obviously can lead to a difference in behaviour. The person may choose to isolate herself and demonstrate general irritability, distractibility, or other responses.

Most autistic individuals are extremely sensitive to even the lightest touch. This is a condition referred to as tactile defensiveness. It is believed that, because the tactile system is working improperly, abnormal neural signals are sent to the cortex in the brain, which can interfere with other brain function. The brain thus becomes overly stimulated, leading to excessive brain activity. The individual cannot turn off this event or organize it. This over-stimulation of the brain makes it difficult for the person to concentrate and may lead to a negative response to touch sensations.[25]

When I was a young child, I would make my arms and legs rigid when my mom attempted to pick me up or hug me. This is quite common, and many mothers of autistic children will tell you of their sadness of feeling "rejected" by their child who does not want to be held or picked up. Not every ASD individual is like this, but the vast majority are! However, there are plenty of ASD children who loved to be hugged and held tightly. Liking to be squeezed tightly is another topic to be discussed shortly.

The most important issue here is to remember to not touch the ASD patient excessively, and minimally at best. Again, as discussed earlier in this book, ask the parent what amount, if any, the patient will tolerate. Don't take it personally if the ASD patient withdraws from your touch.

Vestibular System

The vestibular system refers to the structures within the inner ear, the semi-circular canals, that detect movement and changes in the position of the head. Dysfunction of this system can manifest in two ways: hyperactive and hypoactive vestibular systems. Some ASD individuals may be hypersensitive to vestibular stimulation and have fearful reactions to ordinary movement activities. This can include going on swings, sliding boards, or inclines of any sort. The person may have difficulty learning to climb stairs or go up hills and will fear uneven surfaces. They may even appear clumsy.[26]

Personal Experience

When I was in elementary school, as part of our physical education curriculum, the teachers had the students do tumbling exercises. I was terrified to tumble over and go upside down. I simply wasn't going to do it. Keep in mind that I wasn't diagnosed ASD until the age of 50. So there I was, with the teacher demanding that I do it just like everyone else. Well, I wasn't having any part of it. The next thing I knew, there were 4 adults surrounding me. Each one was grabbing different parts of me—my ankles, shoulders, my head. They all began forcing me into the position to tumble. My feet were pulled apart, my head was being forced down, and I began screaming. They were yelling "come on, Anita, just roll over!" If anyone has ever seen *How the Grinch Stole Christmas*, they will recall that moment when the Grinch suddenly developed the strength of ten Grinch's to hold the sleigh loaded with everything from Whoville. Well, in that moment, I suddenly developed the strength of ten people and sprung myself free of them all and ran out of the room. Of course I ended up in the principal's office, and my mom was called to the school. But at least I never had to tumble. Just imagine that whole scenario happening in today's world of litigation.

To contrast that event, as an adult, I became an internationally published military aviation photojournalist. I got to fly in an F-15 fighter jet, flying upside down and the whole nine yards! I also had to first go in a machine called the multi-seat spatial disorientation device (MSSDD), affectionately known to pilots as the "spin and puke device." I LOVED the MSSDD! I asked to go in a second time. They looked at me as if I were crazy. I couldn't get enough of it. However, I will admit to a case of reverse peristalsis as a result of flying in the F-15.

There is also a hypo-reactive vestibular system. With this, an individual may actively seek very intense sensory experiences to continuously stimulate his vestibular systems. This might include body whirling, jumping, and/or spinning,[27] or even flying upside down in a fighter jet!

Proprioceptive System

The proprioceptive system comprises the components that enable a person to have a subconscious awareness of the body position. This includes muscles, joints, and tendons. It automatically adjusts the body to different situations when functioning correctly. For example, it allows a person to sit correctly on a chair or step into a bus. It also enables the use of fine motor skills such as writing with a pencil, buttoning up a shirt, or tying laces on a pair of shoes. When there's dysfunction, the person can be clumsy, easily fall, have odd body posturing, lack body awareness, eat in a sloppy manner, and have difficulty dressing and buttoning shirts or tying laces. Not surprisingly, the person will demonstrate a resistance to new motor movement activities. A toddler with this disorder might not want to crawl.

Praxis, or motor planning, is another aspect that will be affected by such dysfunction. Praxis is the ability to plan and execute different motor tasks. When functioning properly, it will obtain accurate information from the sensory systems and then organize and interpret the information in order to process the demand. Obviously, if the system isn't functioning at full capacity, the person will have great difficulty attempting an activity.

Implications

Dysfunction within these three systems manifests itself in many ways. An ASD individual can be over- or under-responsive to sensory input. His activity level may be unusually high or unusually low. They might be in constant motion or fatigue easily. It is not uncommon for the individual to fluctuate between these extremes. As stated earlier, when these three systems are not functioning properly, the ASD person will likely have gross and/or fine motor coordination problems. This could also result in speech/language delays and in academic under-achievement. In ASD children, you might also see behavioral issues such as impulsiveness, distraction, and general lack of planning. When confronted with new situations, such children may react with frustration, aggression, or even withdrawal.[28]

Personal Experience

In my younger days, I rode horses in jumping competitions and also was into ice dancing, both sports which necessitated extreme motor control. My instructors for both interests would get extremely frustrated with me because I was completely uncoordinated. During a lesson, I was totally unable to do what they'd tell me to execute. But then, once home, I'd go over and over in my mind the sequence of movements, until in my mind I could fully perform the task. Then, at the next lesson, I'd be able to demonstrate the activity perfectly. This would totally perplex the instructor. They'd ask why couldn't I do it "just like everyone else." Of course, at the time I didn't know that I'm on the autism spectrum. I only knew what worked for me, which was the visualization process I somehow figured out how to use.

The five senses, sight, hearing, touch, smell, and taste, all provide data to an individual for processing. A person with ASD will obviously experience the world around him very differently due to the dysfunction in one or more of these senses. There are even more venues for sensing the environment. These include temperature (thermoception), pain (nociception), and balance (equilibrioception).[29]

How an ASD individual experiences pain will be discussed in Chapter 9. This will be critical for the healthcare provider to understand what to look for.

In conclusion, in the ASD individual, the brain seems unable to balance the senses appropriately, leading to sensory integration dysfunction. Additionally, the brain is unable to filter out background stimuli yet incorporate what is necessary. Thus, the person typically has to deal with overwhelming amounts of sensory input day and night.[30]

You should now have a good understanding of what an ASD individual experiences in her daily life. Hopefully this changes your perception, by seeing the clear picture of why we react to everyday situations in a manner typically different from the rest of the population. I'd also like to add that, because we have to constantly cope with massive sensory overload, it is exhausting in addition to overwhelming. Especially when confronted with new situations, we can rapidly become fatigued.

Footnotes

24.   www.autism.org.uk/sensory

24-a. https://spectrumnews.org/features/talking-sense-what-sensory-processing-disorder-says-about-autism/

25.   https://www.autism.com/symptoms_sensory_overview

26.   https://www.autism.com/symptoms_sensory_overview

27.   http://www.autism.com/symptoms_sensory_overview

28.   https://www.autism.com/symptoms_sensory_overview

29.   www.udel.edu/~bcarey/ART307/project_4b/

30.   www.autism-help.org/comorbid-sensory-problems.htm

Chapter 7
Adaptation to
the Environment

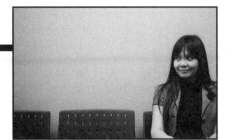

As a health care provider for the past 33 years, I know very well what the environments are of every area of a hospital and various other health care venues. From waiting areas to exam rooms and treatment areas, most areas are generally brightly lit with fluorescent lights. There are typically smells of disinfectant cleaning solutions or other unusual or malodorous smells. There are lots of people, possibly TVs playing, and generally controlled chaos! There are overhead announcements frequently occurring for medical personnel, pagers, and phones ringing. In waiting areas, there are typically many people cramped into seats that are right next to each other. People are milling about, leafing through magazines, using their cell phones, playing noisy games on their phones, and staff calling out patients' names for various reasons. Everyone reading this has most likely been to a physician's office or been a patient at one time or another.

I will propose this question: with the description I just listed above, how were you affected by all of that, if at all? Were you totally aware of all that is going on around you? Probably not. Having read Chapter 6 ("Sensory Issues"), you can now understand that the ASD patient is experiencing all of that to a far greater degree than you. First, the simple fact of being in this environment indicates that the ASD patient is out of her routine. That in itself is typically overwhelming. Second, now being surrounded by an overwhelming array of stimuli coming at her from all directions, the individual can easily reach the meltdown level of sensory overload. Dealing with meltdowns will be addressed in Chapter 9.

The first step to take when you know a patient is ASD, or you suspect him to be, is to take him to a quiet room that's got dim lighting if at all possible. This will greatly diminish the amount of stimuli affecting him. Any type of lighting will be fine, as long as it's not bright, although fluorescent lights can be very bothersome to an ASD person. In any case, make the lighting dim.

A room where there are no other patients or family members present would be best. Be sure to bring along whomever the ASD patient has accompanying him. Being around strangers is very distracting and stressful to the ASD person. The fewer people who are around him, the better.

Try to limit the number of staff members who will be coming in contact with the ASD patient. Don't make it a revolving door of nurses or other ancillary staff. Be sure there is only one person at a time talking to the patient. If possible, turn off cell phones and/or pagers to decrease the possibility of distraction while interacting with the patient.[31]

If there are any sudden noises in the area, such as carts being rolled by or others talking, stop talking to the ASD patient until the distraction has passed. The patient will not be able to focus on what you are saying while there is a secondary source of stimuli in progress.

Color also has an effect on the ASD patient. Warm earth tones would serve well to act as soothing, as would something like a waterfall. Investing in a few small things will be big factors in the effect on the patient. Also, soft chairs or sofas with soft textures would suit her well.

Try to plan ahead and designate a specific room where future ASD patients and their family members may be taken. This way, when such a patient does come along, she can be immediately taken to that area. This will serve well not only for the patient, but also her family and the health care team as well. What that ASD patient experiences upon arrival to a healthcare facility will determine her response as the visit continues. Planning ahead will help ensure a positive outcome for all involved, especially for the ASD patient.

Footnotes

31.   www.medscape.com/viewarticle/840671_2

Chapter 8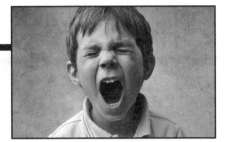

Meltdowns & Safety

An autistic meltdown is quite different from an ordinary temper tantrum. While a typical child might throw a tantrum in order to embarrass or upset a parent with the goal of getting his own way, children with autism rarely have the "mind-reading" tools to intentionally manipulate another person's emotions. The autistic meltdown occurs from sensory overload, which becomes overwhelming to the ASD individual. Meltdowns can occur not only in autistic children, but autistic adults as well. There are typically warning signals given off by the individual which indicate that a meltdown is imminent.

Originally, the word "meltdown" was created to describe what happens when the core of a nuclear reactor is exposed to the air. A series of incidents and warnings lead up to that critical point. Once that happens, it is a major crisis, and lethal exposure to radioactivity occurs or there is a massive explosion. This term embodies the emotional crisis involved in a personal meltdown.[32]

When signs of an impending meltdown begin to surface, it is possible to intervene before the meltdown begins. For example, within the context of this book, an example is given of an ASD patient in a busy emergency department, with bright lights, many people sitting in close proximity, loud noises, and staff scurrying about. All of those stimuli will most likely lead to a meltdown. The simple solution is to get the person to a quiet, dimly lit room with no distractions. Hopefully that will happen before the person is overloaded.

If a meltdown does occur, the ASD person can become overwhelmed by his own emotions. He may stomp his feet, yell, scream, burst out crying, possibly hit others, or self-abuse. This can be extremely frightening to those around the ASD patient, as he might be a large adult who is very strong. The safest thing to do for all involved is get the person to a quiet place. That may necessitate several people to help move the ASD patient.

Thus, it is clear that having a quiet zone readily available for ASD patients to immediately be taken to upon admission is very important. It is much wiser to prevent a meltdown than have to deal with one in progress.[33]

As always, safety is the first priority for everyone involved and others in the area.

Meltdowns may also result from the ASD individual getting fatigued. The more exhausted the person becomes, the more likely she is to suffer a meltdown. Panic, anxiety, rage, or aggression may result from a meltdown, no matter the age of the person.

Dr. Temple Grandin, the most famous autistic person in the world, describes her responses to sensory stimuli like "tripping a circuit breaker." One minute she was fine, and the next minute she was on the floor "kicking and screaming like a wildcat." Dr. Grandin also states that two things she hated as a youngster were washing her hair and dressing to go to church. She has overly sensitive skin and a very tender head. Washing her hair actually causes pain to her scalp. The petticoats that her mother made her wear to church felt like "sand paper scraping away at raw nerves." Of course, Temple would react to these noxious stimuli with tantrum-like behaviors, now referred to as meltdowns.[34]

Another reason an ASD individual might have a meltdown would be due to her routine being changed in some way, especially without any advanced notice. Because of the dysfunction of their sensory processing, she prefers everything to remain exactly the same from day to day. When there's a disruption of her routine, the change, no matter how small it is, becomes intensified to her, and a meltdown might be inevitable.

How to Recognize an Impending Meltdown

An ASD person might begin to display signs of agitation, anxiety, anger, or rage. This could include but not be limited to pacing, hand flapping, fidgeting, crying, screaming, or yelling. There are also physical symptoms that begin to surface. These include rapid heartbeat, flushed cheeks, rapid breathing, cold hands, and muscle tension.

As mentioned earlier, tiredness can also be a trigger for a meltdown. Additionally, hunger and sickness can also lead to disaster. When the person is running on lower emotional or physical resources to cope with situations, the more likely it will result in a meltdown.[35]

It should be mentioned here that a meltdown is far different from a temper tantrum. A tantrum usually results from a child wanting something that is being denied. It is a pure act of manipulation and may involve screaming, punching, throwing themselves on the floor. It is an attention-seeking behaviour. Neurotypical children enjoy to do this out in public because their behaviour will be seen by more people. They will actually use the social situation to their advantage. A tantrum will immediately resolve when the situation is resolved. For example, if the child threw a tantrum because she wanted an ice cream cone, the moment the cone is handed to her, the tantrum stops. Everything will then return to normal.[36]

How to Handle a Meltdown

Before discussion commences about handling a meltdown, it should be stated that it's best to divert one before it happens! A word of thought is to ask the parent/support person who is accompanying the ASD patient what might ignite a meltdown in that person. Always remember to involve those people in the care of the ASD patient.

Here are tips to remember if a meltdown begins, whether it's a child or adult:

- Don't try talking to the individual. Your words and voice will only serve as more stimuli to the person. It will not comfort him.
- Don't touch him. Again, it would only be adding more stimuli.
- Don't try to reason with him.
- Give him some time—it can take a while to recover from an information or sensory overload.
- Once the meltdown appears to be diminishing, calmly ask him (or his parent/support person) if he's OK. Keep in mind that he'll need more time to respond than you might think.

- Simply do whatever you can think of in the environment you are in to minimize sensory overload for the ASD patient.[37]
- Never take personally whatever the ASD patient is doing. His behaviour has nothing to do with you.

Safety

Safety is of course paramount to the ASD patient and everyone around her. Because a meltdown can become physically volatile, it is of extreme importance to have the person in a room with minimal objects that may serve to be picked up and thrown. If at all possible, utilize a room which does not have glass windows or doors, which an angry fist or foot might go through.

Also, it is best for staff to remain clear from the person until the meltdown passes. Avoiding injury is the top priority during a meltdown, for everyone involved.

Personal Experience

As a child, I'd have meltdowns during which my mom would get me dressed in clothing that felt scratchy to me. I'd pull off the item, she'd put it back on me, I'd pull it off, and finally I'd burst out crying hysterically. At that point she would put something else on me, but only after the crying was done and I'd calmed down.

As an adult, my meltdowns are a bit more subdued, but they still can happen. It can result when I'm already stressed over one thing, then something else pops up to add even more stress. Then it's like the straw that broke the camel's back, and I'll burst into tears. It then just has to run its course, typically 5-10 minutes. Once I'm calmed down, I can think more clearly and be better able to handle the situation.

Footnotes

32. https://www.verywell.com/what-is-an-autistic-meltdown-260154
33. https://www.verywell.com/what-is-stimming-in-autism-260034
34. www.myaspergerschild.com/2009/07/temper-tantrums-and-meltdowns-in.html

35. www.myaspergerschild.com/2009/07/temper-tantrums-and-meltdowns-in.html

36. www.autism-causes.com/the-meltdown.html

37. www.autism.org.uk/about/behaviour/meltdowns.aspx

Chapter 9
Pain Perception
of the Autistic Individual

Pain is defined as an unpleasant sensory and emotional experience associated with actual or potential tissue damage or described in terms of such damage.[38]

Pain sensitivity is composed of somatic sensory perception and a subjective emotional reaction, and it plays a key role in warning people to avoid dangerous situations.

There are limited studies that have been done on the pain threshold of ASD individuals. Of the few available, there appear to be differing results. It is known, however, that ASD people, whether children or adults, do demonstrate abnormal responses to painful stimuli. Some people can tolerate extreme heat, cold, or pressure and seem relatively insensitive to pain. Paradoxically, they may experience intense pain from idiosyncratic sources but struggle to communicate it.[39]

A closer look at the literature confirms that, although some people with autism are insensitive to pain, others are unusually vulnerable to it. Sensory sensitivities—exaggerated reactions to certain sounds, lights, touch or other stimuli—affect most ASD individuals. Pain may emanate from autism-related health issues such as gastrointestinal problems. Additionally, difficulties with sleep, anxiety, and perseveration (the tendency to fixate on a particular thought), all common features in people with ASD, may intensify pain.[40]

There are numerous ways an ASD patient might let you know he is in pain. Here's a list to keep in mind:

- He may verbally tell you
- Sign language
- Handwritten note
- Typed note
- Tablet or iPad type device
- Texting from phone
- Pictures or symbols
- Pointing/gesturing
- Pictures with words
- Making sounds
- Crying
- Facial expressions (frowning, etc.)
- Hitting or hurting himself
- Hitting or hurting others
- Other [41]

Tips on Communication

- Recognize that many autistic patients may have difficulty with self-report of symptoms of illness, injury, and pain
- You need to ask the right questions
  - Does something feel different, weird, or uncomfortable?
  - Is something bothering you?
  - Can you show me where it is?
- Be creative.
- Recognize that nonverbal cues (e.g., body language) may not match verbal information.

- Allow for alternative ways of communication other than spoken language (e.g., writing, sign language, texting, use of tablet or other such device, etc.).

- Allow patients (whenever possible) to complete written information on forms before medical visits.

- Allow parent/support person to assist the ASD patient in communicating pain.

- If the ASD patient is able to fill out forms, allow extra time.[42]

Inability to observe and diagnose pain in the ASD patient may lead to late diagnosis, inappropriate treatment, distress, and further disability, and possibly even death.

I read a story a while back about a little boy in the UK with ASD. He was nonverbal, about 4 years old. He'd been displaying symptoms of pain for over 24 hours. His parents took him to the local hospital's Emergency Department. The child was evaluated by the ED physician. The child did not appear to be in any great distress and was discharged home with a diagnosis of stomach virus. Later that night, the little boy died. An autopsy revealed a ruptured appendix. This is a very sad story that may have turned out differently if several things were handled differently. As I read the full account, it appeared that the healthcare providers felt the parents were over-reacting about their son's pain level. Because the child was at the ED, he wasn't acting in the typical manner he routinely did at home. In the ED, he was extremely quiet and non-responsive to the exam. The parents told the staff multiple times that at home he was displaying pain. Of course, what they saw was a quiet little boy who appeared in no distress. Had they understood autism and the not-so-typical ways they might display pain and listened to the parents, the little boy probably would have been evaluated and worked up properly and might still have been alive today.

Personal Experience

In 1982, I was ice dancing and had a bad fall on the ice. As I hit the cold surface, I heard a loud snap. As I got up from the ice, I realized my left arm was fractured, as my hand was literally dangling down when I lifted my arm to a horizontal position. I wasn't feeling any pain. I was annoyed, however, about the impending inconvenience of having a cast on it for the next eight weeks. I walked into the office located in the lobby of the ice arena. I politely asked if anyone could get me to the hospital. They asked why. I had been holding my fractured wrist "together," and I held up my left arm for them to see. When my left wrist dropped down, everyone started screaming at the sight of it. I thought their reaction to be quite funny, and I started laughing. I felt no pain! They summoned an ambulance for my ride to the hospital.

Footnotes

38. https://www.annals-general-psychiatry.biomedcentral.com/articles/10.1186/s12991-016-0095-1

39. https://spectrumnews.org

40. https://spectrumnews.org/features/deep-dive/unseen-agony-dismantling-autisms-house-of-pain/

41. https://redcap.partners.org/redcap/surveys/?s=e2wykW

42. www.painweek.org/education_posts/pain-and-autism-clinical-traits-sensory-perceptions-and-practice-tips.html

Chapter 10
Preparing the Autistic Patient for an Exam or Procedure

I can't think of anyone who's ever said they enjoy going to a doctor's office or hospital for any type of exam or procedure. It is typically an anxiety-provoking event, even for neurotypicals. For the autistic patient, this discomfort is greatly magnified. There are numerous things that can be done to prevent or minimize over-stimulation for this patient population.

Gathering in advance all available information about a patient such as cognitive function, verbal ability, and medical history is a must.[43] A pre-visit phone call with the parent or caregiver is an excellent way to gather all necessary information about the autistic individual. Some hospitals are now doing this to aim for a smooth visit at their facility. That phone conversation could mean the difference between a challenging encounter or a smooth visit. It must be noted here that such an interview should be conducted in a closed, soundproof office, and all data should be entered immediately into the patient's electronic chart. This is in compliance with the Health Insurance Portability and Accountability Act (HIPAA).

There are numerous questionnaires already in use to gather information from the parent or caregiver/support person. Below are examples of the information gathered:

1. Patient's name, age, diagnosis

2. Is he/she verbal or non-verbal?

3. What triggers his/her anxiety?

4. Can you determine when a meltdown is imminent?

5. How does he/she feel about being touched?

6. How does the person communicate (verbally, using pictures, writing, computer device/texting, sign language)? How shall we communicate with him/her?

7. Does the patient avoid eye contact or close proximity with others?

8. What is his/her favorite food and drink?

9. Describe past visits for health care—what might work better this time?

10. Is the patient receptive to visual aids such as a video of the procedure?

11. Does he/she have any phobias or fears?

12. What should be avoided?

13. What are his/her favorite toys/comfort objects?

14. What is the best way to comfort the individual? [44]

Stressors that will arise during a health care visit would include:

1. Overstimulation – Bright lights, over-crowded waiting rooms, loud noises, fast-paced environments, TVs, or music.

2. Unfamiliar environment

3. Long wait times

4. Changes in the patient's routine

5. Unwanted touch—Getting vital signs taken, exams, blood work, procedures [45]

Get the Parent(s)/Caregiver Involved

It is typical for parents of autistic children to be extremely involved in their children's care and life. Healthcare providers should capitalize on this fact and bring the parents on board before the appointment. There is a lot they can do at home prior to the day of the visit.

When a patient with autism is scheduled to come in for a visit, here is a list of things to share with the parent that they can institute at home beforehand.

1. The parent must tell the autistic individual that he will be going to a doctor's appointment or for whatever kind of appointment it is. Depending on the age of the person and his level of understanding, give as much information as possible. Explain why the visit is necessary.

2. If possible, bring the ASD patient to the facility prior to the actual date of the appointment to familiarize him with the place.

3. Book the appointment as the first or last one of the day to minimize wait time.

4. Book a double appointment for the extra time that will probably be necessary.

5. Let the parent know if the healthcare facility has an online portal for autistic patients that may have visual aids, photographs, or videos that will help with the visit.

6. If the ASD patient is young, using dolls to demonstrate a procedure can be very helpful.[46]

7. Tell the parent to bring along the ASD patient's favorite toy, blanket, or security object.[47]

8. Take care of all the paperwork prior to the visit.

9. Suggest that the parent perform role-playing with the ASD patient at home to simulate the exam or procedure.

10. Have the parents prepare a list of questions they want to ask during the visit.[48]

11. If the ASD patient is an adult coming by herself, suggest the following to her:
    - If she has never been to the facility before, she might come and visit prior to the day of the appointment. This will familiarize her with the facility and how to get there.
    - Have her pick up all necessary paperwork prior to the appointment, or have it all mailed to her. It is best to have it all filled out ahead of time. It is one less stressor for her to deal with on the day of the exam.

- Have a pre-visit phone call to discuss the appointment. Answer her questions. You will probably need to ask her if she has any questions or concerns. Be very calm and patient. ASD people tend to not be comfortable talking on phones.

- Instruct her to bring a list of any medications she is taking.

- If any type of lab work is necessary, instruct the ASD patient to be NPO, explaining that this means to not eat or drink after midnight the night before the appointment.

- Suggest that she bring along a book or something else to occupy herself while waiting.

- Tell her that, when she arrives, she will be taken to a quiet room to minimize sensory overload.

- Remind her to bring along a government-issued ID card and her insurance card.

- Suggest she bring sunglasses, headphones, or whatever she typically uses to block sensory input.

- Tell her the staff is knowledgeable about autism and they are prepared for the visit.

Preparing the Staff

The focus is to guard against sensory overload. Simple steps can be taken to decrease or eliminate sensory overload.

1. The first step is to have a designated room that's dimly lit and away from the waiting area that has minimal furniture or medical equipment in it. Upon arrival, take the ASD patient and whoever is with him to that room. If possible, he can be in a room with no other patients or family members. No music should be playing; it should be just a quiet room with no stimuli.

2. Limit the number of staff that will be dealing with the ASD patient. The fewer, the better.

3. Ensure that all staff members who will be caring for the ASD patient is aware of the upcoming visit and that they have been educated about autism and will follow the autism protocol the facility has outlined.

4. Conduct a meeting of staff that will be involved to review the ASD patient's chart and plan of action.

5. If a pre-appointment phone call has been made to the parent, discuss how staff will communicate with the patient.

6. Alert the staff to talk directly and to the point. Don't talk excessively or joke around. Communicate your intentions clearly and directly. Tell the patient what will happen next and why. Maintain a clear sense of structure throughout the visit.[49]

Preparing the ASD patient for the exam is a team effort among the health care providers and the parent/support person. Initially it may seem like a lot of effort, but after the procedure has been followed by a few patients, it will become routine for the health care providers. The positive results they will see will be the reward for their efforts.

Footnotes

43. http://www.acpinternist.org/archives/2008/11/autism.htm

44. http://www.todayshospitalist.com/index.php?b=articles_read&cnt=731

    http://www.acpinternist.org/archives/2008/11/autism.htm

45. https://www.texaschildrens.org/departments/autism/preparing-your-child-autism-hospital-visit

46. http://www.autism.org.uk/about/health/doctor.aspx

47. http://dbptraining.stanford.edu/5_Tutorial/readingdocs/asd_and_surgery_012914.pdf

48. http://autismandhealth.org/?a=pt&p=detail&t=pt_hc&s=hc_prep&theme=lt&

49. http://www.acpinternist.org/archives/2008/11/autism.htm

Chapter 11
The Importance of Websites, Videos, and Albums

Many people with autism benefit from some advance familiarity with new places and procedures. Many are visual thinkers and most effectively process new things by seeing pictures that tell a story. The use of illustrated stories about procedures, surgery, and anesthesia are excellent ways to prepare the ASD patient. Studies and anecdotal evidence have shown that children with ASD are better able to process visual tools than verbal communication.[50]

Under a method called Social Stories, developed by Carol Grey (carolgraysocialstories.com), social stories are used to prepare children with ASD for new and unexpected experiences. Her highly effective proactive method is supported by research. Carol's method is very extensive, and she creates all styles of Social Stories aimed at the varying needs of ASD individuals. For the purposes of this book, the version which uses photos with first-person captions was referenced. A Social Story can be created for the following:

- Visit to doctor's office
- Getting blood work drawn

- Getting vital signs taken

- Monitors such as blood pressure cuff, pulse oximeter, EKG

- Pre-op evaluation

- Getting ready to go to the operating room

- Meeting with the anesthesia provider

- Going to the operating room

- Induction of general anesthesia

- Waking up from anesthesia

- Going to the recovery room

- Leaving to go home

- Stopping at a favorite restaurant on the way home for a treat

- Arriving at home

Other Social Stories include:

- Getting an MRI

- Getting an EEG

- Getting an ultrasound

- Radiology/x-ray

- Angiogram/Cardiology

- Speech and language therapy evaluation

- Audiology

It is most effective for the ASD patient to review the Social Story as far in advance as possible prior to the event. That allows him ample time to process the information and review it as many times as he'd like.[51]

When creating each Social Story, the following are some suggestions to remember:

- Include an introduction, body, and conclusion

- Answer who, what, when, where, and how

- Write it in first person (as if the ASD patient is telling the story)

- Use positive language to describe responses and behaviors

- Make sure it is literal and accurate

- Use concrete, understandable words to go with the visual supports

- There should a photograph for each step with the brief caption

- Use a style and format that is motivating [52]

An example of this would be a Social Story about being in the pre-op area. There should be only two people in the photos, a nurse and the patient.

1. The first photo would be of the patient standing in the pre-op area, next to a chair, with a big smile. In the background is the monitor. The caption would state something like "Wow! I'm here to get ready for surgery! I feel very brave today!"

2. The second photo is of the patient sitting in the chair with the BP cuff on, the pulse oximeter on their fingertip, and EKG hooked up, again with a big smile. The nurse is depicted leaning over as if she is tending to the pulse oximeter. The caption could read, "This is fun to learn how my heart beats! It doesn't hurt. Just lots of wires hooked up on me!"

3. The third photo would be the patient, having changed into the hospital gown, smiling. The caption would read, "I'm now in a special gown! It feels fine to wear it!"

4. The fourth photo is of the patient lying on the gurney with the head of the bed upright, waving at the camera, smiling. She can be holding her teddy bear or favorite blanket, with the nurse standing at the bedside. The caption could read, "I'm so happy that I can bring Teddy to the operating room! And mom can walk down the hall with us!"

You get the picture. Each photo is simple, depicting the patient as being happy and not scared. Captions are minimal and positive. This will give the ASD patient an excellent idea of what will happen in the pre-op area. If possible, when making your Social Stories, use the actual staff that will be taking care of the patient in the photographs. A familiar face goes a long way in comforting the ASD patient.

These Social Stories can be posted on the health care facility's website using a link specially designed for ASD patients. By having these available on a website, the ASD patient and his family can access it at any time and look at them multiple times. The same Social Stories can be used in an album at the facility in each department where procedures would be done and in the pre-op area as well. For the albums, laminated pages that can be removed to stay with the patient for comfort can also be utilized.

Short videos of the same scenarios can also be made available on the website and at the facility. If the facility has a special waiting area for ASD patients (as hopefully it will), the videos can be watched in that area.

Very young children with ASD or those who are not yet using words or phrases will not be able to follow the Social Stories. The use of FIRST/THEN cards should be employed. The "First" is the non-preferred activity, and the "Then" is the preferred activity. An example of the "First" would be a photo or illustration of a doctor looking into a child's ear with an otoscope. The "Then" photo is the child eating a cookie. They will understand that first the undesirable event will happen, but it will immediately be followed by a desirable event.[53]

Again, these FIRST/THEN cards should also be included on the website as well as available on site.

Lastly, it would be a good idea to provide several age-appropriate items that the ASD child may select to entertain herself. Examples could be squishy toys, coloring books and small packs of crayons, colored pencils, and little note pads in case the ASD child wants to draw or write something. These items would then be given to the child to keep. They are all inexpensive items that can be purchased in bulk. The cost of them far outweighs the comfort it will bring to the child, keeping them entertained and distracted from where he is.

Using a Power Point template, it will be very easy to create your own Social Story of your health care facility and for each department that an ASD patient might need to visit. The Social Story should actually begin with a photograph of the outside of the building and of the entrance they will be coming through. There can be photos of the path to the admissions desk, the person behind the desk, the process of signing in, getting the little name bracelet placed on his wrist, getting into a wheelchair to be transported to the pre-op area, etc., depicting every step of the way. By the time the ASD patient finally arrives for his appointment, he will feel as if his has already been there. That will go a VERY long way in giving him a feeling of peace, comfort, and security.

Footnotes

50.   http://dbpeds.stanford.edu/content/dam/sm/neonatology/documents/asd_and_surgery_012914.pdf

51.   http://www.rchsd.org/documents/2015/03/autismspeakstoolkit.pdf

52.   http://www.rchsd.org/documents/2015/03/autismspeakstoolkit.pdf

53.   http://www.rchsd.org/documents/2015/03/autismspeakstoolkit.pdf

Chapter 12

Identification of Autistic Patients

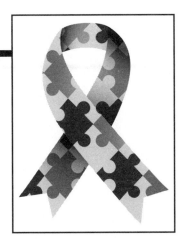

The puzzle ribbon was adopted in 1999 as the universal sign of autism awareness. Although this image is a trademark of the Autism Society of America, the organization has granted use to other non-profit organizations in order to demonstrate unity and advance a universal mission.[54]

The Autism Society of America defines the Autism Awareness Ribbon as follows: The puzzle pattern reflects the complexity of the autism spectrum. The different colors and shapes represent the diversity of the people and families living with the condition. The brightness of the ribbon signals hope that, through increased awareness of autism and through early intervention and access to appropriate services/supports, people with autism will lead full lives, able to interact with the world on their own terms. This is the most recognized symbol of the autism community in the world.[55]

Admission to any healthcare facility is the appropriate time to identify the individual as being ASD. Obviously, permission must first be granted from the individual or the parent/support person accompanying her to have the symbol of the Autism Awareness Ribbon identifying her as being on the autism spectrum. In today's arena of litigation and HIPAA regulations, it is recommended that a printed document concerning this matter be available and signed by both the patient/family member/support person along with a witness from the medical staff. This is the same procedure used for a consent form for surgery and anesthesia. This will put the healthcare facility in the clear of any future issues regarding the identification of the autistic patient.

Upon admission to a hospital or ambulatory surgical center, each patient dons the traditional wristband. This contains the patient's medical record number, the date, their name, and possibly a few other details. For the ASD patient, a sticker of the Autism Awareness Ribbon could be added to the wristband.

If the ASD individual is going to a doctor's office for a routine appointment, the Autism Awareness Ribbon sticker can be placed on the chart or somewhere within the paperwork. For confidentiality purposes, perhaps the sticker should not be on the outside of the chart. This also means, however, that other healthcare providers then might not be made aware of the patient's ASD. It should be up to each facility to determine how to notify all those involved in the care of the ASD patient, while still maintaining his privacy.

Most likely you will find that the ASD patient and his family/support person will be so happy that the staff understands autism and demonstrates that extra attention will be given to him. In any case, it all needs to start at the admissions desk or sign-in area and continue with the patient until his final discharge.

Footnotes

54.   www.autism-society.org/about-the-autism-society/history/autism-awareness-ribbon/
55.   www.autism-society.org/about-the-autism-society/history/autism-awareness-ribbon/

Chapter 13
Emergency
Department

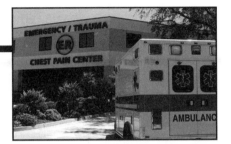

For patients with ASD, the emergency room can be so overwhelming that it undermines their ability to get the treatment they need. ASD individuals use the emergency room just as much as others, if not more so. This is especially true for ASD adults who tend to not seek regular health care; when something becomes a health crisis, they head to the nearest ER. By this point, their anxiety is high, and they are much more likely to suffer a meltdown. Beside the operating room suite, the ER is a place where the training of the entire staff can make all the difference between a negative outcome and a positive experience. The training needs to include everyone from the check-in receptionist to the discharge person and everyone in between.

It is readily evident that parents and staff members get frustrated with the frequent behavioral escalations that ASD patients experience while in the ER and the team's inability to effectively prevent or manage these situations. The medical team also recognizes that failure to manage the behavioral escalations interferes with timely and optimal medical care.[56]

Through the research for this book, it was discovered that a small but growing number of hospital ERs are implementing accommodations for the ASD population. These changes include offering calming objects like toys and iPads and sending patients to quieter areas that are dimly lit. While this certainly is a positive step in the right direction, much more needs to be done to provide effective care for the ASD patient.

A health care facility that implements complete autism training, such as that which this book offers, will attract ASD patients to its facility. This is a financially wise decision for hospital administrators to consider. Once it became known in a community that a hospital is autism-friendly and has staff trained about autism, of course every ASD patient will flock to that facility for his health care.

ER experiences have been very traumatic for ASD patients and their families when staff members are inexperienced and lack knowledge about autism. Except for the time necessary to train staff, there is minimal to no cost to a health care facility to institute this service to their patients.

What a Parent Can Do

Many individuals with ASD have multiple medical problems, such as epilepsy or GI issues, leading to frequent visits to the ER. Parents can help to prepare their child for a visit to the ER by talking to her about it and also taking her to see the ER ahead of time. This advance planning can surely help to ease the stress when the time comes to visit for care.

The parent can also inquire at the ER if any visual supports are available, such as an online source for ASD patients. It is extremely helpful for every health care facility to have such a site available that parents or adult ASD patients can access that offers videos and photos of the facility, procedures, and staff. By seeing all this ahead of time, the patient's stress level will be decreased because it will be familiar to the ASD patient once she arrives at the facility.

Most parents of ASD patients are already advocates for their child. Parents can call ahead to the ER to alert the staff that they are bringing in their autistic child. They can also advocate for him in the ER to alert staff about how the ASD patient will be able to communicate with the staff. The parent can also request a quiet room to wait in that's dimly lit. The parent can also bring along a favorite cup in case any oral medications might be given, a favorite blanket or toy, or whatever routine item the ASD patient would like.[57]

Ways the ER can best serve its ASD Patients

1. At the admissions desk, once it is known that the patient checking in is ASD, the first step should be to take the ASD patient and whoever is accompanying her to a designated autism room. The room should be quiet

with dim lighting. There shouldn't be any other patients or families in the room, just some comfortable seating. It should be in an area set apart from the noise and chaos of the ER. The health care facility should designate a specific room for this purpose. Not only will it serve as a comfort zone for the ASD patient, but it should also alert the staff to adjust their communication style and institute the autism protocol. Don't take anything personally, such as the ASD patient being loud, disruptive, or unpleasant. Keep in mind that the patient is out of his comfort zone in an extremely high-stress environment.

2. Once in the "Autism Room," all intake information can then be obtained in privacy. The admissions desk employee can first come in to get the basic information required of all patients such as the reason for the visit, demographic information, and of course insurance information. At this point, it can be determined how the ASD patient will be able to communicate with the staff. The triggers for the ASD patient must also be determined in addition to any special information the staff should know about the ASD patient. The ASD patient's diet should be obtained in case he is on a special diet. Sleep patterns are also important in addition to any special therapies. Parents of these children often seek alternative medicine for their child. While all this must be respected, such treatment could have detrimental effects on the child that the parent isn't aware of.

3. Next, the staff member such as a nurse or physician's assistant, will obtain the health history of the ASD patient from either the parent, caregiver, or from the patient themselves. It is best to include the ASD patient in the conversation. Don't talk about her as if she is incapable of comprehending what you are saying.

4. It is imperative that the number of staff that will be involved in the patient's care be extremely limited. Each new person entering that room will be yet another stressor to that ASD patient. She is already in a heightened state simply by being there in the ER. Each of these staff members must be thoroughly educated about autism and how to effectively deal with the ASD patient.

5. Keep the conversation to a bare minimum in a low, calm voice. Don't use any small talk or try to be cute or initiate conversation with the ASD patient. Excess words only serve to increase sensory overload. When talking to the ASD patient, use very simple questions that can be answered with a yes or no. Too much wording can overwhelm and confuse him.

Ask what he would like to be called, and use that name when talking to the ASD patient.

6. Prior to obtaining the ASD patient's vital signs, the equipment can be offered to him to look at and touch. This will help to lessen his stress level and give him a chance to ask any questions he might have about the equipment.

7. Maintain patience. Appointments with ASD patients will surely necessitate more time. However, consider that if they are not given the time they need to process everything, it can rapidly spiral downward, which could take a whole lot longer.

8. Once all the basic information is obtained as well as vital signs, the ASD patient will need to be transported to the exam room. Tell her what will be happening. State calmly and clearly that she will be taken to an exam room, either by wheelchair or stretcher, whichever is necessary. Inform her that the exam room will be more brightly lit and they will be passing other patients, staff, and possibly noisy areas along the way.

9. The ER should have disposable sunglasses available, like those given out at ophthalmologist's offices after patients' eyes are dilated. Offer a pair of these sunglasses to the patient to protect her eyes from all the bright lights that will be encountered along the way to the exam room and for once in the exam room. Those rooms tend to be brightly lit to enable the attending staff to see a wound or for examining a patient or doing a procedure.

10. The ER should also have available at least one set of earphones with disposable covers for the patient if they want to drown out the loud noises inherent to a busy ER.

11. The ASD patient's parent/caregiver must be allowed to accompany him to the exam room. There should also be an exam room designated at the end of a hall or farthest from the nurses' station to minimize noise.

12. Try to minimize the wait time for the ASD patient in both the initial waiting room and then for the exam and any treatments. The longer the wait time, the higher her anxiety will go.

13. During the actual exam, the staff member should first tell the ASD patient exactly what he is going to do, as briefly as possible. Let the patient see the stethoscope or any devices to be used during the exam. Let him touch the items and process what he is seeing.

14. Minimize touching to a bare minimum. In general, autistic individuals don't like to be touched, even by family members, let alone strangers. Don't attempt to hug them, pat them on the back, or even shake their

hand. All of that only serves to heighten their anxiety level.

15. If any lab work is ordered or tests such as MRIs or x-rays, the decision for any sedation might arise. Of course, it's best not to sedate the ASD patient and instead proceed with calm communication. The parent is your best source to state what has worked in the past for successful management. If the ASD patient already has an IV, than Versed can be administered via the IV. If not, the oral route can be used. Even when seeing an adult ASD patient, think about using oral Versed mixed with juice or something to mask the taste. Keep in mind that many autistic individuals have food aversions and might be reluctant to drink anything unless it tastes like a special drink. If the parent brings his favorite cup, all the better! Chapter 14 ("Inpatient Admissions") discusses sedation of the ASD patient in more detail.

16. Stimming—If the ASD patient chooses to use some sort of fidget toy or device throughout the exam, she should be allowed to do so, unless there is a reason not to do it. That is how she is dealing with her anxiety. Trying to make her stop will only agitate her or increase her already high level of anxiety.

17. Explain why any tests are necessary. Videos or photo albums of any procedure are helpful at this time to show the ASD patient. He will do much better to know exactly what will be taking place.

18. If the ASD patient needs x-rays or anything done outside of the ER, it would be best if the staff member accompanies the patient to the area and stays with him throughout the test/procedure. The parent/caregiver should also be allowed to come along for support.

19. In an optimal health care setting, ALL staff will be educated about autism so they can provide continuity of the care the ASD patient received in the ER.

20. It is best to expedite any tests, lab work, and medications to greatly reduce wait times.[58]

21. Never assume an ASD patient is not listening if he is not responding. He may just be overwhelmed and unable to respond. Also, never think he is having a temper tantrum. If he gets to the point of a meltdown, it isn't bad behaviour—it's an overload of sensory stimulation he no longer can cope with. Refer to Chapter 8—Meltdowns to better understand how to deal with this situation, should it arise.

22. If the ASD patient is not to be kept NPO, she should be offered something to drink.

23. Keep the ASD patient and her parent/caregiver informed of what's going on, including updates on wait

time. She will greatly appreciate frequent updates rather than sit there not knowing what's going on.

24. Before a test or procedure is done to the ASD patient, it should be demonstrated on a doll or even on the parent/caregiver. Allow the patient time to process the demonstration. The ASD patient can even "assist" in the demonstration process.

Conclusion

All health care staff members need to understand autism in order to properly treat this rapidly growing population. Additionally, health care providers must utilize the ASD patient's parent/caregiver as their best resource person. No one knows the ASD individual better than the parents do, and their input will be the most valuable tool to optimize care for that patient. Through education and collaboration, the ER visit for the ASD patient can be a positive experience.

Footnotes

56. https://www.childrenshospitals.org/newsroom/childrens-hospitals-today/issue-archive/issues/fall-2014/articles/managing-patients-with-autism-to-effectively-deliver-care

57. https://www.autismspeaks.org/blog/2012/08/03/reducing-anxiety-er

58. http://www.baynews9.com/content/news/baynews9/news/article.html/content/news/articles/cfn/2016/2/8/nemours_emergency_ro.html

Chapter 14
Inpatient Admissions

In order to have a successful, positive inpatient admission, there must be a comprehensive, coordinated, multidisciplinary team approach for the ASD patient, whether a child or an adult. This includes but is not limited to the following specialties:

- Pediatricians/Internal Medicine/Family Practice
- Child/Adult Psychiatrists/Psychologists
- Neurologists
- Nutritionists
- Specialists in gastroenterology, metabolic, and sleep disorders
- Therapists, counsellors, other specialists[59]
- Social worker/Case manager
- Speech and Language pathologists
- Occupational therapist

This entire model must also be family centered along with the above multi-disciplinary team effort. The family knows the ASD patient the best, and their input will be invaluable. This allows for family-centered decision-making regarding the care of the ASD child/adult. You can strive to improve autism health care through high-quality, data-driven, evidence-based health care.[60]

Intake Forms for Inpatient Admissions

Each health care facility needs to create an intake form for the parent(s) or other support person of the ASD patient to be filled out upon admission. Of course, if the ASD adult patient can complete the form himself, allow him to do so. This gathering of information will provide the foundation upon which the care plan can be developed for the ASD patient.

Below is an Autism Care Questionnaire that can be adapted to each facility. Permission to use this form was granted by the Lurie Center for Autism, MassGeneral Hospital/Mass General for Children.

Autism Care Questionnaire

Patient Information

Date: _____

Patient's name: _____

Patient's date of birth: _____

Patient's current age: _____

Name of person completing this form: _____

Relationship to the patient: _____

Email address of the person completing this form: _____

Communication

1. How does the patient like to communicate his/her needs/wants? (Check all that apply)

   - ❑ Talking
   - ❑ Sign language
   - ❑ Typed words
   - ❑ Handwritten words
   - ❑ Tablet or communication device
   - ❑ Pointing/gesturing

   - ❑ Pictures/symbols
   - ❑ Pictures with words
   - ❑ Making sounds
   - ❑ Facial expressions (smiling, frowning, etc.)
   - ❑ Other

2. What other ways will the patient tell us what he/she wants/needs? (Check all that apply)

   - ❑ Talking
   - ❑ Sign language
   - ❑ Typed words/handwritten words
   - ❑ Tablet or communication device
   - ❑ Pointing/gesturing

   - ❑ Pictures/symbols
   - ❑ Pictures with words
   - ❑ Making sounds
   - ❑ Facial expressions (smiling, frowning, etc)
   - ❑ Other

3. How does the patient communicate "yes" or "no" when asked a question? _____

4. How does the patient learn new information or instructions? (Check all that apply)

   - ❑ Talking
   - ❑ Sign language
   - ❑ Typed words
   - ❑ Handwritten words
   - ❑ Tablet or communication device
   - ❑ Stories

   - ❑ Pictures or symbols
   - ❑ Pictures with words
   - ❑ To do/finished boards
   - ❑ First/Then boards
   - ❑ Other

5. How does the patient know that time is passing? (Check all that apply)

   ❑ Using a clock or watch
   ❑ Using a timer
   ❑ Using schedule boards
   ❑ Counting aloud
   ❑ Other

6. What is the best way for us to prepare the patient for tests? (i.e., how long the wait will be or how long the test will take?)

   _____

7. How will the patient tell us that he/she has to go to the bathroom?

   _____

8. How will the patient tell us that he/she is hungry or thirsty?

   _____

9. How will the patient tell us if he/she is in pain? (Check all that apply)

   ❑ Talking   ❑ Making sounds
   ❑ Sign language   ❑ Crying
   ❑ Typed words   ❑ Facial expressions (frowning, etc.)
   ❑ Handwritten words   ❑ Hitting or hurting self
   ❑ Tablet or communication device   ❑ Hitting or hurting others
   ❑ Pointing/gesturing   ❑ Other
   ❑ Pictures or symbols

10. Are there other ways the patient will let us know that he/she is in pain? How?

   _____

The Hospital Visit and Exam

1. How should we greet the patient? _____

2. What is the best way for us to examine the patient?

   ❑ Communicate with the patient (using the favored communication method) before each step of the exam
   ❑ List or count things that the doctor needs to do, i.e., look in the eyes, look in the ears, listen to the heart
   ❑ Do parts of the exam on someone else first to demonstrate
   ❑ Allow the patient to touch any instruments used (i.e., blood pressure cuff, stethoscope, pulse oximeter, thermometer)
   ❑ Hide instruments until they become necessary
   ❑ Distract the patient during the exam
   ❑ Other

3. Is there a part of the exam that may especially bother the patient? (Check all that apply)

   ❑ Using a stethoscope to listen to the lungs   ❑ Looking in mouth/throat
   ❑ Checking blood pressure with the cuff   ❑ Belly exam
   ❑ Eye test   ❑ Testing reflexes
   ❑ Ear test   ❑ Other

4. Will the patient wear a hospital gown? _____Yes _____No

   If no, what will the patient want to wear? _____

5. Will the patient wear a hospital ID band on his/her wrist? _____Yes _____No

   If no, please let us know before coming to the hospital, as all patients must wear an ID wristband.

Comfort and Safety

1. What is the patient sensitive to? (Check all that apply)

   ❑ Loud noises   ❑ Specific colors   ❑ Touch
   ❑ Unexpected noises   ❑ Fragrances/smells   ❑ Specific types of touch
   ❑ Bright lights   ❑ Textures   ❑ Other

2. How long does the patient sleep at night? _____

3. Will a family member or caregiver be staying with the patient? _____Yes _____No

   If yes, what hours will the person be at the hospital?_____

4. Are there any special ways to make mealtime easier? _____Yes _____No

   If yes, what? _____

5. Is the patient on a special diet? _____Yes _____No

   If yes, what type? _____

6. Are there special times of the day that the patient eats snacks or meals? _____Yes _____No

   If so, what are they? _____

71

7. Does the patient prefer that different foods in a meal not touch or to have separate plates for each food item? ____Yes ____No

If yes, what does the patient like? _____

8. Are there any words, phrases, or actions that will upset the patient? _____Yes _____No

If yes, what are they? _____

9. How will he/she let us know that he/she is anxious/upset? (Check all that apply)

❑ Talking
❑ Sign language
❑ Typed words
❑ Handwritten words
❑ Tablet or communication device
❑ Pointing/gesturing
❑ Pictures/symbols

❑ Pictures with words
❑ Making sounds
❑ Facial expressions (frowning, smiling, etc.)
❑ Physical motions (rocking, flapping, squeezing hands)
❑ Hitting or hurting self
❑ Hitting or hurting others
❑ Other

10. What comforts the patient when he/she gets upset or anxious? (Check all that apply)

❑ Talk to him/her
❑ Leave him/her alone
❑ Give him/her some space
❑ Other

11. What may help decrease the patient's anxiety? (Check all that apply)

❑ A map of the hospital
❑ Low lighting
❑ Sunglasses
❑ Headphones to decrease noise
❑ A heavy blanket

❑ An escort that will help the patient around the hospital
❑ Music
❑ Videos
❑ Puzzles/games
❑ Other

12. Are there any other safety concerns we should know about? _____Yes _____No

If yes, what are they? _____

13. Is there anything else we should know so we can make the patient's visit as positive as possible?

_____

Accommodations

When an ASD patient must undergo an inpatient procedure in a hospital, it would be best to provide a private room. Most hospitals seem to be making that possible for all patients, but it should happen in particular with this patient population. If the ASD patient has to be in a room with another patient, he could face massive sensory overload from the presence of the other patient. The other patient might want to watch the television all the time, talk on the phone, people coming to visit and so forth. It will be enough sensory overload for the ASD patient to be in a private room, so he doesn't need more to stress him out. He is there to heal, and it is up to the staff to optimize the patient's environment and comfort.

Another reason it is critical that the ASD patient be admitted to a private room is that the staff can accommodate the parent/support person to stay with him at all times. It is a major stressor to the ASD patient to be out of her home in unfamiliar surroundings. There is always a lot going on at a hospital that will cause the ASD patient to get overwhelmed. If the door is open to her room, all the activity in the hallway can be over stimulating. It is also best if possible to provide a room as far away from the nurses' station as possible. That is where there will be around the clock noise from conversations, people coming and going, phones ringing, and other sources of endless noise.

Today, hospitals are providing sleeper sofas or hide-a-beds in the private rooms. The parent/support person can then stay there with the ASD patient. In addition to providing emotional support, the parent is present to participate in decision-making with the health care providers. This is a win-win situation for everyone.

Staff Caring for the ASD Patient

As part of the team effort, a list should be generated of staff members who will be taking care of the ASD patient. Limit the number of personnel who will be involved. Mary Didie, M.D., a pediatric attending at Blythedale Children's Hospital in Valhalla, N.Y., says she not only tries to limit the number of physicians and staff who treat an autistic child, but she also works to use the same nurses and assistants whenever possible.[61]

Dr. Erich Maul, D.O., a pediatric hospitalist at Kentucky Children's Hospital in Lexington, is the father to an 8-year-old boy with autism, and is somewhat of an expert on treating children with autism. He agrees with the notion of limiting the number of physicians, nurses, and other staff who will care for the ASD patient. This can be a problem at academic centers where attendings often enter the room as part of "a huge galloping hoard" of residents and medical students. When doctors insist on rounding with their entire group of residents, he explains, "some of these kids are going to act out." He also states, "They frequently have disruptive behaviors such as screaming or physically acting out." Dr. Maul says, "Doctors need to realize that socially unacceptable behaviour can be normal for children with autism."[62]

All staff involved should always remember that they must plan to spend more time with the ASD patient. They can't expect to rush in and out repeatedly. Again, it must be noted that parent/support person involvement is extremely important. However, even in a quiet room, parental guidance and knowledgeable staff might not be enough to entice the ASD patient to cooperate. Fortunately, medical advances have given hospitalists some alternatives to sedation. There are more ancillary services for inpatients than in years past, including pediatric psychologists and child-life specialists. Such advances have led to "a recognition that we can use other strategies than sedation," says Dr. Michelle Marks, the head of pediatric hospital medicine at Cleveland Clinic Children's Hospital.[63]

Most of these parents have a great deal of experience with physicians and tend to be more hospital-savvy than the average parent. "They know their child well and want to participate in their child's medical care," says Dr. Marks from the Cleveland Clinic. "They are the only ones who know what is normal for their child. If you're smart, you're going to utilize them to your advantage."[64]

It must be noted that, when risk outweighs benefits, a procedure must be aborted. If an ASD patient gets out of control, simply stop and let her calm down. If the test is necessary to make a diagnosis, then it will need to be rescheduled. Physicians must fight the urge to forego necessary tests and procedures. Dr. Drake in Dallas notes that, because colleagues have passed on difficult exams, she has seen missed ear infections, abscessed teeth, and other problems that could have been easily treated. "It's a difficult balance between providing comprehensive care and making patients more anxious," says Dr. Drake.[65]

Nutrition

There are several feeding problems related to autism. The most common feeding problem associated with autism is selective or restrictive eating whereby a child consumes a very narrow range and number of foods. It is estimated that 60-89% of autistic children are selective eaters. Foods are often refused due to texture, smell, or even the plate it's served on! Parents of these children are aware of all of these complicating factors. Almost two thirds of autistic children eat fewer than 20 foods.[66]

It must be noted here that autistic children might have difficulty swallowing, GERD, or other gastrointestinal problems. Whether it's just one day, a week, or longer in the hospital, the ASD patient will need a menu plan that accommodates their special needs. Of course, the parent/support person will be of tremendous value in this arena. They may have already brought along a special plate. Depending on the reason for the admission, there may be a special diet prescribed by the attending physician. This will be more challenging to get the ASD patient to eat an unfamiliar meal. Where possible, it is best to maintain the patient's normal diet. The parent will best know how to handle the situation.

Sedation of the ASD Patient

Children with ASD have a range of medical problems involving many organ systems. A subset of children with ASD has abnormal mitochondrial energy production and function that contributes to their physical, cognitive, and behavioral impairments. The presence of mitochondrial dysfunction increases the risk for potential damage to the brain, which is dependent on oxidative metabolism.[67]

Anesthesia and sedation do not present a problem for most children with ASD. However, ASD children with mitochondrial disturbances are at increased risk for the following potential complications:

1. Excessive time to emerge from anesthesia

2. Developmental regressions—These could include loss of expressive and/or receptive language, gross motor skills, fine motor skills, cognitive function, and overall neurologic deterioration. In some children, skill loss may be permanent.

3. Excessive fatigue and reduced energy levels: temporary (for days or weeks) or persistent.

4. Possible death.

Chapter 18 will provide more in-depth information about anesthesia for the ASD patient.

It should be noted that benzodiazepines inhibit adenosine nucleotide translocase, which is necessary for mitochondrial functioning. Propofol is also known to inhibit mitochondrial functioning.[68]

When sedation is necessary, it is imperative to gain knowledge about the ASD patient's triggers and sensory issues, states Laura Badwan, M.D., hospitalist site leader for the pediatric intensive care unit at Children's Memorial Hospital in Chicago, who also works on the sedation team. "Talk to the patient's families to assess their autistic traits and find out what has worked best in the past," Dr. Badwan says. For example, if the ASD patient has an oral aversion, then you should steer clear of trying to give oral medications. Dr. Badwan also offers several tips for sedation of the ASD patient:

- Encourage the parents to talk to their child about the test or procedure.

- Try to stick to the ASD patient's normal routine. Maybe schedule the sedation close to nap time.

- Bring a favorite cup or toy with the patient to the sedation area.

- Bring the patient to a quiet room for the sedation and for after the sedation to recuperate in.

- For ASD patients, who don't have an oral aversion, consider oral Versed in their favorite cup for IV placement. These patients might get combative during IV placement. A little Versed goes a long way in calming them down. In addition, Dr. Badwan points out that Versed has amnestic properties, so the patient won't remember anything.

- Keep in mind that some autistic patients may get more combative after sedation. The decision should be discussed ahead of time regarding whether to give more sedation or abort the procedure.[69]

Safety

The healthcare team must determine the likelihood of the ASD patient to express aggression or physical violence or make active attempts at leaving the area.[70]

Transitions

The ASD patient must be allowed extra time when transitioning from one place to another. If possible, take the person to the pre-op area the day before their surgery to see the place ahead of time, or simply when going from their room to MRI or the lab, etc. Just go slowly. Give him time to adjust from one place to another.

Small Talk is a Big Deal!

Most non-autistic people engage in small talk. ASD individuals typically don't, and it's best to NOT engage in it with them or in their presence! It will only act as sensory overload and could even result in a meltdown! They are already stressed out, and coming in their room chattering away about the weather might be the straw that breaks the camel's back.

In conclusion, a multidisciplinary team approach to care is essential for the inpatient ASD patient. This demonstrates the need for all health care providers to have a solid working knowledge of autism and best practices in caring for this rapidly growing population. A positive outcome for the ASD patient also means a positive outcome for all the staff.

Footnotes

59.   https://www.autismspeaks.org/science/resources-programs/autism-treatment-network/what-atn

60.   https://www.autismspeaks.org/science/resources-programs/autism-treatment-network/what-atn

61.   http://www.todayshospitalist.com/index.php?b=articles_read&cnt=731

62.   http://www.todayshospitalist.com/index.php?b=articles_read&cnt=731

63.   http://www.todayshospitalist.com/index.php?b=articles_read&cnt=731

64.   http://www.todayshospitalist.com/index.php?b=articles_read&cnt=731

65.   http://www.todayshospitalist.com/index.php?b=articles_read&cnt=731

66.   http://www.bradleyhasbroresearch.org/Feeding_Problems_Common_in_Children_with_Autism_/

67.   http://www.mitoaction.org/files/Risk%20of%20Anesthesia%20Regression%20(2).pdf

68. http://www.mitoaction.org/files/Risk%20of%20Anesthesia%20Regression%20(2).pdf

69. http://www.todayshospitalist.com/index.php?b=articles_read&cnt=731

70. https://www.childrenshospitals.org/newsroom/childrens-hospitals-today/issue-archive/issues/fall-2014/articles/managing-patients-with-autism-to-effectively-deliver-care

Chapter 15 Preparing for the Operating Room

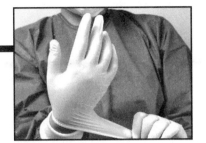

The prospect of going for surgery and anesthesia is daunting for anyone, even more so for the ASD patient. I have been working in the operating room for the past twenty-eight years. Being autistic, I see it through the same eyes as an ASD patient. There are countless sources of stimuli that the patient will be confronted with. Imagine an ASD patient being wheeled into the operating room, with the bright glaring lights and a scrub tech slinging heavy metal trays loaded with surgical instruments, making harsh, stinging, loud sounds. Whenever I encounter an autistic patient, I immediately institute my own "autism protocol" that I get my co-workers to go along with. I've been doing this for over six years now, at which time I got diagnosed with autism. All the things I do are simply instinctive based on all my own sensory issues and autistic ways. Now I want to take this to a global scale.

Health care providers will encounter autistic patients, whether they are children or adult patients. They may know ahead of time or at the time of the ASD patient's appointment. When the staff is educated about autism and a plan is in place, there is far greater likelihood that the outcome will be optimal for the ASD patient. Autistic individuals have an invisible disability. Blind people use a white cane with a red tip, and physically disabled people use a wheelchair. Their disability is readily seen by everyone. For the autistic patient, there is nothing that is seen by others. What complicates matters for health care providers is the broad range of disorders on the autism spectrum. People might see a ten-year-old child who's non-verbal with great limitations of communication, and the next one might be a high-functioning autistic adult who's very adept at communicating. Despite the level of functioning, each ASD patient has the same sensory issues and processing delays of varying degrees. In the perioperative setting, everything becomes greatly magnified, and any coping skills will dramatically decompensate. It is up to the health care providers to enable themselves to be ready to successfully handle the next autistic patient they encounter.

Hospital administrators must look at the growing population of autistic individuals and realize the importance of taking the necessary steps to best prepare their staff for this need. During the research for this publication, it was discovered that a small but growing number of hospitals are beginning to recognize that they must educate their staff about autism. They are implementing new strategies to care for this unique population. Not only must the health care providers be prepared, but all ancillary staff must be as well. From the secretary at the admissions desk to the patient's final discharge, everyone must know how to successfully handle the ASD patient.

Child Life Specialists

Many health care facilities are now utilizing Child Life Specialists (CLSs) who are brought into cases with ASD patients. These CLSs work closely with children and families, providing emotional support. They also help develop family coping strategies. With a background in child development, psychology, and counseling, CLSs help explain medical jargon to kids and prepare them for surgery or procedures.[71]

A CLS would also need to be specially trained in caring for autistic patients.

When the ASD Patient Needs Surgery or Anesthesia for a Procedure

The perioperative needs of the ASD patient differ in every way from the neurotypical patient. Both the behavioral and metabolic needs must be met for both a safe and successful visit to the operating room. It is suggested that each facility devise its own autism-friendly anesthesia care plan, adjusting it to meet the needs of each ASD patient. It would be best to minimize the number of drugs administered to these patients. Some of them may have underlying mitochondrial disorders, so there are certain drugs to avoid for this population. The ability of the health care team to be flexible and creative will determine their ability to care for this unique group of patients.

From the very start, it must be recognized that ASD patients are challenged by new surroundings and a change in their routines of daily life. Before the actual day of surgery, there is much that can be done ahead of time to prepare the ASD patient.

It is recommended that each facility designate a pre-op room specifically for its ASD patients. The room must be dimly lit, away from the noisy chaos of the nurses' station, and the room can be closed off to minimize noise. Limit the amount of equipment in the room. Also, limit the number of staff that will be caring for the patient. In fact, the pre-op nurse should accompany the ASD patient to the operating room when it's time to go there. That will provide the ASD patient with a sense of peace and security. Also, the parent should be allowed to walk with the patient as far as possible. Some facilities allow the parent to change into scrub attire, hat, and mask and allow him or her into the operating room to be there until the ASD patient is asleep, and then the parent is escorted out of the OR and back to the waiting area. Wherever that is possible, it is highly recommended.

It must also be remembered that ASD patients' ability to communicate might decompensate in times of stress such as being at the health care facility. Staff must remember to continue talking to the ASD patient despite her looking down or away and probably turning expressionless. Staff must also remember not to take any of this behavior personally. Just understand this is how an ASD individual copes with anxiety and stress. Remember to stay calm and use a calm voice when talking. Limit your wording, using very short, direct sentences. Allow the ASD patient to feel she is part of the process. Give her choices whenever possible. Keep the parents directly involved. They are your best source of information to keep things going smoothly.

Key Point

There must be a highly coordinated effort among all staff for the ASD patient, and their autism protocol must be instituted. This will facilitate the continuity of care necessary for a smooth and successful outcome for the ASD patient.

1. Parents are encouraged to discuss the upcoming surgery with their ASD child, whether the individual is a child or adult. They can explain why the surgery or procedure is necessary. If age/level of understanding is appropriate, they can use a doll the show the child what body part will be affected. Even if the child doesn't appear to be listening, parents should proceed to provide an explanation.

2. The ASD patient can be brought to the facility for a tour to see the pre-op area and meet the staff who will be caring for him on the day of surgery. It will also help the ASD patient to go to the facility the day before if it on a route he is not familiar with. Driving him there and back home will serve to familiarize him with roads he's never been on before. If there's a restaurant along the route that the ASD patient enjoys, point it out that on the day of surgery they will stop there on the way home afterwards! Also, if a pre-visit does occur, the ASD patient can be given a disposable head covering and disposable booties to take home to play with. That will help acclimate the patient to seeing everyone wearing those items on the day of surgery.

3. The health care facility should conduct a phone interview with the parent prior to the day of surgery. The Autism Care Questionnaire from Chapter 10 can be utilized for this purpose. Information on the ASD patient's mobility, communication methods, likes, dislikes, and phobias are an absolute minimum requirement. Of course, the patient's entire health history and previous surgeries is a necessity. Find out about his previous experiences, what worked, and what didn't. Also, establish any medications the ASD patient might be taking. Such drugs could include stimulants, anti-psychotics, or bedtime melatonin. These could affect anesthesia.

4. The health care facility should consider a web site for ASD patients to visit prior to their surgery. This website would provide a step-by-step pictorial of what the patient will experience upon arrival. It would start out with a photo of the front of the facility, going into the entrance, the admissions desk, the pre-op area. Then would be photos of the basic equipment in pre-op, such as the blood pressure cuff, pulse oximeter,

EKG wires, and sticky patches; the pre-op nurses who would be caring for him; photos showing a pediatric patient having changed into the hospital gown; and a patient on a stretcher, with the nurse at the bedside and the patient's favorite stuffed animal under his arm. Show an IV being placed in patient's hand. Show the patient being wheeled down the hall to the operating room with the pre-op nurse and parent walking beside and the patient's stuffed animal coming along. Show the patient with the anesthesia provider showing her a mask, going into the OR with a view of the overhead lights and the operating table. Show the patient meeting the OR staff who will be assisting the surgeon and the staff putting the mask on the patient's face. Then show the recovery room and a nurse caring for the patient. Show the patient's parent/caregiver there in the recovery room with him. Show the patient ready to leave in street clothes, as a transport person pushes him in the wheelchair. Everyone is smiling and waving goodbye as the patient is leaving the hospital. Show the patient getting into the car with the parent/caregiver. Show them stopping at the patient's favorite restaurant for a treat on the way home. Show the patient back at home with a big smile.

A picture guide such as this should portray the patient and everyone in the photos with happy faces. The ASD patient can look at these photos as many times as she want. It will serve to make her feel comfortable once she is at the health care facility, as she will feel she has been there before. What might seem silly to a neurotypical person actually is a big deal to an autistic individual!

5. Enlist the help of the ASD patient at home prior to the date of surgery in packing things for the big day. Have him select a favorite item he wishes to bring along, such as a teddy bear, doll, or blanket. Have him pick out a favorite cup which can be used if sedation will be given. Tell him ahead of time that he might need to drink something special once at the hospital. If sedation is given, it will serve not only to calm the ASD patient but also to provide amnesia for the event as well.

6. Parents must explain to the ASD patient that he will not be able to eat or drink anything after midnight for the day of surgery. They can explain that it is for his safety to have an empty stomach. Follow that with a statement that, on their way home, they can stop at his favorite restaurant for a meal.

7. Schedule the ASD patient's surgery or procedure as the first case of the day. That will minimize the waiting time, thus limiting the stressors to the patient.

8. Staff must remember to offer support to the parents/caregivers of the ASD patient. The whole peri-operative experience places a lot of stress on them as well, and they must not be forgotten. A kind hand on their shoulder, reassurance of taking excellent care of their ASD child, keeping them updated on progress, and possibly offering a hot or cold beverage will go a long way.

9. There is increasing evidence that some individuals with ASD have biochemical and metabolic abnormalities. These may include mitochondrial dysfunction, increased lactate, general B-vitamin complex deficiency, and increased oxidative stress associated with membrane lipid abnormalities.[72]

    Although anesthesia and sedation do not pose a risk for most children with autism, a small number of these children suffer unpredictable regression in skills and behavior with such treatment. It might simply be prudent to adopt a suitable anesthetic plan for all ASD patients in general, thus avoiding any post-operative complications. Recommendations include good hydration, minimal fasting, use of normal saline instead of lactated ringer's (due to elevated blood lactate levels), maintenance of good body temperature, acid-base balance, and avoidance of oxidative stress.[73]

10. If the ASD patient is young enough to get an inhalation induction, then the IV can be secured after she is asleep. If not, then an IV must be started in the pre-op area. Elicit help from the parent if the child has seen the online video of this aspect. If not, then approach the matter differently than you would with a neurotypical patient. If the child has her teddy bear with her, you can demonstrate starting the IV on the bear. If not, ask the parents if it is OK to use them as the demonstration model. Explain each step as you go. Be sure to use Emla cream or whatever local anesthetic cream your facility uses when preparing to start an IV. Some ASD patients may require sedative premedication to alleviate anxiety and promote cooperation with the preoperative phase. This is where good communication with the parent and staff can facilitate the ASD patient to willingly drink the mixture of medication and some liquid in their favorite cup. Although Midazolam is a commonly used sedative, in some ASD patients, it may cause them to become paradoxically dysphoric rather than sedated. Additionally, Midazolam can inhibit adenosine nucleotide translocase, which is necessary for mitochondrial functioning. For this reason, Lorazepam is often used in this setting in low doses.[74] As with any medication, the user should verify any and all side effects and determine the

correct dosage for each patient.[75] Patients taking regular medication to modify their behaviour must be taken into consideration on an individual basis.

11. While in the pre-op area, the anesthesia provider should bring a mask for the patient to play with prior to going to the OR. The provider can show the ASD patient how to put it on her face and tell her that the mask will help her to sleep. Avoid using terminology like "We will put you to sleep." ASD individuals take things literally and may have had a pet that was put to sleep. They will think you mean they will be euthanized. Once she has the mask on her face, tell her to practice blowing up a balloon. This may have to be demonstrated with a real balloon!

12. Remain alert to the signs of the ASD patient's anxiety increasing and heading towards a meltdown. Information should have been obtained from the parent/caregiver ahead of time as to what are triggers for the patient and the signs the patient begins to display when her anxiety is increasing. Safety must always come first for both the ASD patient and staff.

13. Once the IV is secured, the ASD patient will be calm, and all necessary staff have interviewed the ASD patient and her parent/care giver, they are then ready to be transported to the operating room. As stated earlier, the pre-op nurse should accompany the ASD patient to the OR along with the OR circulating nurse or anesthesia provider who is transporting the patient to the OR on the stretcher/gurney. This new staff member should have already come to the pre-op area earlier to introduce themselves to the ASD patient and their parent to familiarize themselves. That again will promote a feeling of comfort and security to the ASD patient. Of course allow the ASD patient to bring along their teddy bear, doll, or comfort blanket. Having a familiar object will again provide comfort and security.

14. Prior to wheeling the ASD patient to the OR, tell her that she will be passing many people, a lot of noise, and people moving very quickly. Explain that this is typical activity for an operating room area. Allow the ASD patient to wear a set of headphones if she has one, or provide one if she doesn't. All health care facilities should have a few of these on hand for this purpose. Also offer disposable sunglasses as well. Be sure to push the stretcher/gurney nice and slowly. Typically, the pace of the whole operating room suite is rush-rush-rush. However, with this patient population, that won't work. Remember to be flexible, creative,

and patient! If the ASD patient received any pre-op medication, be sure to wait until it has taken effect before embarking on the journey to the OR. Remember not to touch the ASD patient except when necessary.

15.   The operating room should have the temperature setting at a comfortable setting, neither too cold nor too warm. The overhead operative lights must be off. A suggestion is to induce anesthesia with the patient on the stretcher/gurney. That would eliminate moving her onto the operating table, thus providing less opportunity for stress or anxiety to increase. Tell the ASD patient what is being done before it happens. For example, say that the pulse oximeter is being put on her finger, the blood pressure cuff on her arm, and the little sticky pads going on her chest. Again, don't touch her any more than necessary. If it's going to be an inhalation induction, let her hold the mask again, like she did in pre-op. Tell her to put it over her mouth and nose and blow up the "balloon." If it's an IV induction, act quickly but safely to get her to sleep. Of course, all monitors must be on and pre-oxygenated. Again, elicit help from the ASD patient in the pre-oxygenation process.

16.   After induction, proceed as usual. The anesthetic drugs of choice will be discussed shortly. It will be suggested here that keeping the anesthetic as simple as possible will promote faster recovery. Good analgesia is essential, with liberal use of local anesthetic techniques. Anti-emetic drugs and an isotonic crystalloid fluid bolus such as normal saline can minimize postoperative nausea and vomiting. These measures are particularly important with the ASD patient. It may be very difficult to distinguish between the potential causes of postoperative distress, pain, nausea, emergence delirium, unfamiliar nurses, or residual disorientation from pre-op sedation.[76]

17.   Once the ASD patient is in the recovery room and is awake and responsive, he has full control of his airway, there are no indicators for need of administration of any medications, and it was straightforward surgery, it might be considered appropriate to remove the IV. That is one less point of distress to the ASD patient. However, if the IV is necessary, wrap the site with something soft and non-constricting to secure the IV site. Have the ASD patient's parent/caregiver present in the recovery room as soon as the patient is brought there. Explain to the parent that the child will probably be very sleepy at first but will gradually awaken. Their presence will be invaluable when the ASD patient sees his parent. Again, limit touching to only what's necessary. The parent can provide suggestions on what will work best for the child.[77]

18. If the ASD patient received a nerve block or some type of local anesthetic injection, the parent must be notified to prevent the ASD patient from injuring the affected area. This should be discussed with the patent and ASD patient ahead of time. Otherwise, the ASD patient might panic that a body part is numb and feels like it's not there.[78]

19. Some institutions are allowing the ASD patient to be discharged home on the day of surgery, sooner than other patients, to minimize the stress of being at the hospital. Typically, a post-op patient must eat, drink, or pass urine prior to being discharged. However, with ASD patients, in order to minimize the disruption in their daily routine, after discussion with the parent on continued care at home and only after the ASD patient has regained his baseline in terms of orientation and mobility, then he can be discharged home.[79]

20. Provide the ASD patient with an explanation that she will be leaving the hospital, and she will be transported to the exit door in a chair that has wheels. Of course, the parent/caregiver will walk alongside her. Ask the parent and ASD patient if they have any questions. Be sure all discharge instructions have been reviewed and are understood. Be sure the parent has any prescriptions for pain management or antibiotics written out by the surgeon.

21. Suggest that the parent stop on the way home and get the ASD patient a treat or small gift from the gift shop for being such a wonderful patient! The parent might be so exhausted by that point that he/she might forget to do this! A friendly reminder will help him/her remember.

22. Thank you for taking such great care of one of my people! Your acts of kindness go a long way.

In-House Therapy Dogs

Some hospitals are recognizing the importance of therapy dogs to provide comfort to their patients. As their name suggests, therapy dogs are trained to provide affection and comfort in therapeutic situations. Typically, they work in hospitals, nursing homes, and other health care facilities.[80]

For any health care facility interested in obtaining one of these dogs, there is an excellent website for reference: http://www.assistancedogsinternational.org.

Therapy dogs are used in the pre-op area for comfort and entertainment for this patient population.

In conclusion, there are many things that need to be done to provide the ASD patient with a successful outcome. However, once these extra actions are taken a few times by the staff, it will become routine. Take pride in yourself for going the extra mile to make a big, positive difference in your patient's life. Even though the ASD patient might not pop a smile at all throughout the visit, the simple fact that he didn't suffer a meltdown tells you it was a positive experience for him. Always remember the quote by Dr. Temple Grandin's mother, Eustacia Cutler, that autistic individuals are "different ... not less."

Footnotes

71. http://health.usnews.com/health-news/health-wellness/articles/2014/07/07/7-facts-about-child-life-specialists

72. Chauhan A, Chauhan V. Oxidative stress in autism. Pathophysiology 2006; 13: 171–81

73. Davi A. Anesthesia and sedation risks in children labeled with Autistic Spectrum Disorder. 2010. Available from http://www.epidemicanswers.org/wp-content/uploads/2010/05/Anesthesia-Risk-in-Children-with-Autism-.pdf (accessed July 2012).

74. http://www.medscape.com/viewarticle/808453_5

75. http://whatmeds.stanford.edu/medications/lorazepam.html

76. http://www.medscape.com/viewarticle/808453_5

77. http://www.medscape.com/viewarticle/808453_5

78. http://www.medscape.com/viewarticle/808453_5

79. http://www.medscape.com/viewarticle/808453_5

80. https://www.autismspeaks.org/blog/2016/07/15/service-dog-or-therapy-dog-which-best-child-autism

Chapter 16
Anesthesia for the Autistic Patient

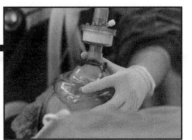

I have been an anesthesia provider for over 28 years at this point in my career. I've calculated that to be over 55,000 cases to date. Throughout my entire career as a Certified Registered Nurse Anesthetist, I've always gone the extra mile for my patients. Sometimes this necessitated using my break time to stay at the bedside and talk to them, providing extra reassurance and comfort. Sometimes it meant dreaming up creative techniques to accommodate a physical deformity or some special need. Whatever it takes to accommodate each patient, I've always been up to the task.

After accidentally discovering I'm on the autism spectrum at the age of 50, I set out to be an autism advocate at the highest level; doing everything I can to enable those on the autism spectrum to lead healthier, happier, productive lives. Each time I encounter an autistic patient, I institute my autism care plan, and without fail, the result is a happy patient and a very happy parent. I've heard many stories from the parents of these kids, of one disaster after another their child had on trips to the operating room. Unfortunately, this patient population has many co-existing conditions that warrant frequent visits to doctors, operating rooms, or simply the use of anesthesia for an MRI.

Whatever the reason for a trip to the operating room, the responsibility rests in the hands of the health care providers to make it a positive, successful, and safe experience. Anesthesia providers must first grasp the concept that autism is an invisible disability. There is no wheelchair or white cane that indicates disability. The reality is that autism can provide significant challenges related to everyday tasks others take for granted. With the rapidly growing number of children being diagnosed on the autism spectrum, most anesthesia providers will encounter ASD patients in their practice. They will also encounter ASD adults, as millions are now just receiving their ASD diagnoses in their 50s, 60s, 70s, and 80s. The children with ASD frequently will be seen getting radiological procedures such as an MRI or CT scan, ENT and dental procedures, or surgery of some sort. ASD adults will most likely be presenting for surgery.

With the unique individual needs and behaviors of this patient population, there will be a challenge to develop an anesthesia plan for ASD patients. Each person with autism has different needs, emotional triggers, and coping skills. The best way to care for these patients is through education about autism and advance planning. The best place to start is with the parents or caregivers. They are with that ASD patient probably more than any parent you will ever meet. They know that child best. It is critical to accept the fact that you need to incorporate their suggestions into your plan of action. Medical professionals in general are not used to having family members directly involved in their patients' care. One must also maintain respect for not only the ASD patient but also the parent(s) or caregivers as well. These parents typically devote every breath to the care of these kids (or adults). They may be trying alternative measures for health care that may seem strange or bizarre to you. They are often desperate measures to try anything to help their child.

Autistic individuals might easily be labeled as difficult patients. You must keep in mind that their behaviors are a result of how they experience the world around them. If an ASD patient has a meltdown, it is a result of sensory overload. This is totally different from a neurotypical individual having a temper tantrum. More information on meltdowns vs. temper tantrums can be found in Chapter 8 ("Meltdowns and Safety").

In order for the anesthesia experience to be a positive one, there must be a very coordinated effort among the entire perioperative team. In addition to the anesthesia pre-operative health history which is obtained for each patient, the anesthesia provider must be provided with the data obtained from the initial autism care questionnaire. This should be reviewed prior to walking into the ASD patient's room in the pre-op area, and preferably a day or two prior to the day of surgery. In order to maintain continuity of care, the actual surgical team must also be involved. In my twenty-eight years as an anesthetist, it's not uncommon that, as a patient is being wheeled into the operating room, the following things are going on:

- The scrub techs are counting instruments and handling heavy metal trays laden with instruments, making sudden, harsh, loud noises.
- Multiple OR staff members laughing and talking loudly about what they did over the weekend.
- Blinding overhead surgical lights are turned on.
- The temperature in the room is turned way down to about 65 to accommodate the staff.
- Music is playing loudly.
- Many people are in the room, like equipment reps, medical students, scrub techs, circulating nurses, the surgeon(s), and anesthesia providers. I look at it as controlled chaos!

With the description above of an operating room, it rapidly becomes apparent that ALL healthcare professionals must receive the information in this book *The Complete Guide to Autism for Health Care Professionals & Ancillary Staff*. The entire OR staff must understand autism and understand why all the measures are being taken as well as be able to plan ahead of what to do and what not to do to make it a positive, stress-free experience for the ASD patient. Additionally, anesthesia providers must understand that ASD patients are not only a challenge from their behavioral standpoint but also from a metabolic standpoint.

ASD Patients with Mitochondrial Dysfunction

The metabolic issues an ASD patient might have affect the choice of anesthesia. Unfortunately, unless an ASD patient has a known history of mitochondrial dysfunction, one cannot differentiate this sub-group from other autistic individuals. Unless the patient goes for mitochondrial genomic analysis, this pathogenicity of mitochondrial oxidative phosphorylation will be undetected.[81]

The presence of mitochondrial dysfunction increases the risk for potential damage to the brain, which is dependent on oxidative metabolism. This risk is more pronounced in procedures that require anesthesia.[82]

In 2003, *The New England Journal of Medicine* published a report by Selzer, et al., on the risks of nitrous oxide in individuals with MTHFR (Methylenetetrahydrofolate Reductase) and concluded, "patients with a diagnosis of severe MTHFR deficiency should not receive nitrous oxide as anesthesia. In the case of emergency procedures, patients whose clinical presentation fits that of severe MTHFR deficiency, even if the disorder has not been diagnosed, should also not receive nitrous oxide. In the case of elective procedures, patients whose clinical presentation fits that of severe MTHFR deficiency should be evaluated, and the diagnosis should be ruled out before anesthesia with nitrous oxide is contemplated." [83]

Risk Factors for Anesthesia Complications

1. History of seizures

2. Respiratory problems

3. Poor health

4. Undiagnosed mitochondrial dysfunction

5. MTHFR gene polymorphism

6. Increased homocysteine levels

7. General B-vitamin complex deficiency or B-12 deficiency (indicated by methylmalonic acid) as cause of homocysteine levels [84]

Experts in the mitochondrial disease field recommend including the following tests on patients with ASD.

1. Comprehensive metabolic profile
2. Magnesium
3. CBC with differential
4. Creatine kinase
5. Amylase
6. Ammonia
7. MTHFR
8. Homocysteine
9. Methylmalonic acid (for B12 status)
10. Fasting glucose
11. Lactate level [85]

Complications That May Occur in the ASD Patient That Has Underlying Mitochondrial Dysfunction

For most individuals with ASD, anesthesia and sedation do not pose an increased risk. However, those with mitochondrial dysfunction are at increased risk for the following:

1. Excessive time for emergence

2. Developmental regressions, which could include loss of expressive and/or receptive language, gross motor skills, fine motor skills, cognitive function, and overall neurologic function. In some individuals, skill loss may be permanent.

3. Excessive fatigue and reduced energy levels: temporary (for days or weeks) or persistent

4. Possible death [86]

Suggestions for Anesthesia for the ASD Patient

Chances are that the anesthesia provider will not be able to order all of the lab work listed above. It might be wise to treat every ASD patient as if he has a mitochondrial dysfunction. This caution relates to the use of universal precautions for each and every patient. You never know which one might have a transmissible disease, so simply protect yourself at all times. The same applies here. The safest approach is simply to do the following:

1. ASD patients should be the first case of the day to limit NPO time (as well as stress of waiting)

2. Avoid nitrous oxide

3. Avoid Lactated Ringer's, since it contains lactic acid, and patients with mitochondrial dysfunction generally have elevated blood lactate levels. Normal saline should be fluid of choice

4. Avoid succinylcholine

5. Maintain normal blood glucose, body temperature, and acid-base balance [87]

6. Be generous with fluid replacement; dehydration is the major cause of post-operative nausea. Instead of administering multiple drugs to prevent nausea, why not simply give the ASD patient appropriate fluid

replacement so they don't have to contend with polypharmacy to metabolize

7. Suggest to the parent of the ASD patient that he take a B-vitamin complex (B6, B12, Folate) a few days prior to the surgery/anesthesia

8. In an article posted on the United Mitochondrial Disease Foundation web site written by leading experts in the field of mitochondrial medicine, Bruce Cohen M.D., John Soffner M.D., and Glen DeBoer M.D., titled *Anesthesia and Mitochondrial Cytopathies*, make the following recommendations for patients with mitochondrial disease:

   • Strict attention should be devoted to respiratory function before, during, and after surgery, especially in patients with abnormal preoperative respiratory signs and symptoms. Vigorous respiratory physiotherapy should be standard postoperative care in patients with pulmonary difficulties. Early use of ventilation and CO_2 elimination should be maintained. [88]

   • Delay elective surgery if any signs of infection are present

The following table was created by Cohen, DeBoer, and Soffner to illustrate the adverse effects of general anesthesia on mitochondrial function: [89]

Medication	Biochemical and Clinical Effects on Mitochondrial Function
Barbiturates	Inhibits Complex I activity at high levels
Benzodiazepines	Inhibits adenosine nucleotide translocase
Propofol	Inhibits mitochondrial function
Halothane	Increased risk for heart rhythm disturbances
Nitrous Oxide	Neurotoxic, possibly by increasing nitric oxide production, which inhibits cis-acotinase and iron-containing electron transport enzymes: affecting energy production
Non-depolarizing agents	Increased sensitivity to the paralytic effects and prolonged responses reported
Local Anesthetics	Bupivacaine uncouples oxidation and phosphorylation

Chapter 16: Anesthesia for the Autistic Patient

Personal Experience

In 2007, I had to have surgery for a rare form of cancer on my right shoulder, called Dermatofibrosarcoma Protuberans. This was prior to my knowing I'm autistic. I underwent the surgery at the hospital I worked at then (and still do), and I had one of the best anesthesiologists provide my anesthesia. My mom was still alive at the time, and they let her come into the recovery room to sit at my bedside. It took me hours to wake up. My mom was getting extremely nervous at how long it was before I even woke up and looked around. I can remember opening my eyes, seeing my mom, the anesthesiologist, one of my co-workers who I was friends with, and a nurse all hovering around my bed, staring at me. I then immediately went back to sleep. A few hours later, I woke up, still in the recovery room, Mom still sitting there. The nurse came over and stated that it was nearing 5:00 pm, and if I didn't get up shortly I'd have to be admitted for an overnight stay. That was a good motivating factor to get me sitting up. The moment I got up, I realized I was so weak I could hardly stand up. My mom helped me get dressed, then two nurses came and helped me into a wheelchair. They wheeled me out to the valet parking area and got me into my truck. My mom drove us home. I remember what a daze I was in. I also recall how weak I was, to the point that I could barely lift my arms or legs or even hold my head upright. Fortunately, I didn't have any nausea. I felt too weak to speak. While in the recovery room I was using head gestures to indicate yes or no. It wasn't until we were home that I attempted to speak. When I did, I was horrified at what I heard. My voice was so hoarse, I sounded like a 95-year-old man. My mother looked at me in shock.

At first my thought was that perhaps I was a difficult intubation, which could explain my hoarseness. I then called the anesthesiologist. He was surprised to hear my hoarse voice. He stated I was a Grade 1 to intubate, and he was very upset at my voice. He was totally perplexed at my condition. So was I. The other thing I was so baffled at was the extreme exhaustion I was experiencing. When we had arrived home, I was able to make it to the couch in the living room. That's where I stayed for the next few days. I simply couldn't get up. Eating and drinking were a chore, and I was only able to eat very small amounts, very slowly. By the fourth day, I was able to get up. I had my surgery on a Friday, thinking I'd be back to work the following Monday. It didn't work out that way. I ended up being off the entire following week. All I could do was lie in bed or on the couch, exhausted. As an anesthesia provider, seeing thousands of patients after surgery, I knew this wasn't a normal way for a body to react to the anesthesia. Now that I know I'm autistic, I don't have to wonder any longer. I obviously have some degree of mitochondrial dysfunction. As for the hoarseness, obviously because my entire body was weak, and so too were my vocal cords, thus explaining the hoarseness. My anesthetic consisted of the following for the 3-hour surgery:

- Versed 2 mg
- Fentanyl 100mcg
- Atracurium 5 mg as a pre-treatment dose
- Lidocaine 100 mg
- Propofol 150 mg

- Succinylcholine 120 mg
- Sevoflurane as aninhalation agent
- Lactated Ringer's as IV fluid
- Zofran 4 mg
- Decadron 4 mg

Now that I know I'm autistic and have some degree of mitochondrial dysfunction, here are the changes I would make to the above list of medications: Normal saline instead of Lactated Ringer's. I wouldn't want to give up the Zofran or Decadron, as I didn't experience any nausea or vomiting. If I'd have had that, I would have been far worse off than I was. I also think that simply the stresses surrounding having surgery and anesthesia contributed to my extreme fatigue. That is stressful to everyone, and even more so to an ASD patient. I'd take a B-complex vitamin with B6, B12, and folate. I'd also take magnesium and vitamin D, both of which ASD individuals are found to be deficient in.

Preparing to Take the ASD Patient into the Operating Room

- Review the ASD patient's Autism Care Questionnaire and discussed it with the entire team that will be involved in the operating room.
- Bring the mask off the circuit when you go to see the ASD patient if it's a child. You can also bring a few choices of fragrance oils for the ASD patient to select one. You may also have her actually put it on the inside of the mask with a Q-tip in the pre-op area.
- Calmly enter the ASD patient's room in pre-op. Introduce yourself. Ask the parents/caregivers how best to communicate with their child. If the ASD patient is an adult, ask him the same question. Be patient.

Remain calm. Don't make any kind of extreme facial expressions. ASD individuals can't read facial expressions so they won't know what you mean, and they might even get upset. Keep your tone of voice soft and pleasant. No extremes with your voice either. Don't take anything personally, no matter what happens! And don't expect your ASD patient to look you in the eye! However, even if she remains looking down, she still hears everything you say. It might take her longer to process it all and to respond, but don't think she isn't paying attention. Don't try to make small talk. Be very direct in what you have to say, and make your sentences short and to the point. ASD individuals take everything literally, so watch what you say! For example, don't use the term "put to sleep." The family dog may just have been put to sleep, and the patient will think she is going to be euthanized!

- Ask if the ASD patient wants to wear headphones on the way down the hall to the operating room.
- Offer a pair of disposable sunglasses to the ASD patient to wear to the operating room to block out the bright lights along the way.
- Tell him that he will be passing many people who will be walking fast and that there might be various sounds as well.
- Tell him that there might be unusual smells as well.
- Discuss with the OR staff that the patient is an ASD patient.
- Shut off overhead surgical lights.
- Have only half of the room lights on.
- Set the temperature at 72 degrees, neither too hot or too cold.
- Have absolutely no music or radio on.
- All instruments must be counted and ready to go. Absolutely no touching of instruments or lifting/placing down of trays.
- Absolutely no testing of bone saws or drills of any sort.
- Instruct everyone not to talk once as the ASD patient is being wheeled into the operating room.
- Instruct everyone not to touch the patient or make small talk with her.
- Be prepared to induce the ASD patient on the stretcher/bed she was brought into the operating room on. Once she is asleep, then everyone can lift her over onto the operating table. That will be far less stressful

than either having the ASD patient move herself over to the operating table or the team lifting the ASD patient over to the table.

- At the conclusion of surgery, while the ASD patient is still asleep, move her from the operating table back onto her stretcher/bed. Because she is still asleep, she won't feel everyone touching her during the move.

- If she came to the operating room with her favorite blanket, be sure that's what is on her, touching her body. Don't put a hospital blanket against her skin, as those blankets are typically rough.

- As patient is emerging from anesthesia, everyone must remain silent, and no one should touch the patient.

- No instruments or metal trays should be handled.

- Be sure to shut off the overhead surgical lights, and have only minimal lights on in the room.

- Once the patient is awake and extubated, very quietly and calmly proceed to the recovery room. Again, no touching. Of course, if it medically necessary such as checking the IV site or something of that nature, then you must do what you need to do with minimal touching.

- In the recovery area, take the patient to the ASD designated room. Give the report to the PACU nurse just as always, being specific that the patient is ASD. The PACU staff should be called ahead of time to alert them that an ASD patient is coming. The ASD patient's parent/caregiver should already be there waiting for the patient to arrive.

- Share with the parents/caregivers everything you did to make the ASD patient's surgical experience a positive one. They will be eternally grateful to you!

It will be literally impossible to determine if your ASD patient falls into the subset with a mitochondrial dysfunction. Simply treat all of them as if they have some form of the mitochondrial dysfunction. Keep their anesthetic as simple as possible, limiting what you give them. Never give nitrous oxide to any of them.

Once you perform these steps a few times, they will all become second nature.

Footnotes

81. https://www.ncbi.nlm.nih.gov/pmc/articles/PMC2584230/

82. http://www.mitoaction.org/files/Risk%20of%20Anesthesia%20Regression%20(2).pdf

83. http://www.mitoaction.org/files/Risk%20of%20Anesthesia%20Regression%20(2).pdf

84. http://www.mitoaction.org/files/Risk%20of%20Anesthesia%20Regression%20(2).pdf

85. http://www.mitoaction.org/files/Risk%20of%20Anesthesia%20Regression%20(2).pdf

86. http://www.mitoaction.org/files/Risk%20of%20Anesthesia%20Regression%20(2).pdf

87. http://www.mitoaction.org/files/Risk%20of%20Anesthesia%20Regression%20(2).pdf

88. http://www.epidemicanswers.org/wp-content/uploads/2010/05/Anesthesia-Risk-in-Children-with-Autism-.pdf

89. http://www.epidemicanswers.org/wp-content/uploads/2010/05/Anesthesia-Risk-in-Children-with-Autism-.pdf

Chapter 17
Women's Health

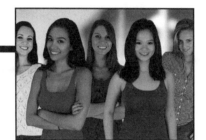

It is only recently that autistic females are gaining the spotlight in the autism world. In the past, it was believed that the ratio of autistic males to females was 4:1. This is no longer seen to be the case.

Health care providers in the field of gynecology and obstetrics must recognize that they will have patients with ASD. Whether it's for general pelvic health, issues with menstruation, pregnancy, or menopause, females with ASD need the same health care just like other females. Due to the sensory issues these individuals face, an examination at an OBGYN's office will most likely cause far more distress than it does your other patients. There are numerous things that can be done to eliminate or lessen the unpleasant steps of the exam.

Another recent advancement for autistic individuals is the acknowledgement that there are millions of autistic adults! Yes, indeed, those autistic children grow up and become autistic adults! There is so much focus on autistic children that it seems to have lost sight of the fact that, once they grow up, the autism doesn't go away. While the CDC reports that 1 in every 68 children are getting diagnosed on the autism spectrum, no one is reporting how many autistic adults there are. There are millions for sure, many of whom are getting diagnosed later in life. The reason for this phenomenon is that the work by Dr. Hans Asperger of Vienna, Austria, didn't get translated into the United States until 1994. By that time, older adults on the autism spectrum were long out of school and simply went under the radar. These individuals thus went through life without any kind of early intervention or services (like me) that are now the mainstay for children getting diagnosed early in life.

Not many females enjoy going for a pelvic exam or a mammogram. The ASD patient can be traumatized by the same visit. There are several factors involved. First, due to developmental disabilities and sensory issues, sensations experienced during the exam could cause a massive sensory overload, causing the patient to have a meltdown. Healthcare providers might forget to think of their ASD patients as sexual beings. It is not uncommon for disabled individuals to be thought of as being asexual. Never assume the ASD patient is asexual, not sexually active, not interested in getting pregnant, not pregnant, or simply does not want to discuss contraceptive methods.

There is one more point to be made, and that is on the topic of sexual abuse of autistic females. People with autism are more likely to be raped or sexually abused. Limited sexual knowledge and experience and social deficits are believed to be some of the variables contributing to this risk, according to S.M. Brown-Lavoie et al at the Department of Psychology, York University, Toronto Canada.[90]

According to the Centers for Disease Control, approximately 1 in 6 boys and 1 in 4 girls suffer from sexual abuse before the age of 18. Additionally, the U.S. Department of Justice's National Crime Victimization Survey, the country's largest and most reliable crime study, reports that, every two minutes, a person is sexually victimized in the United States, and the numbers regarding individuals with disabilities are even higher.[91]

While no specific numbers exist for individuals with autism, research suggests that this population is extremely vulnerable to being sexually abused.

Dr. Shana Nichols, clinical psychologist, founder of the ASPIRE Center for Learning and Development, tells Autism Speaks, "Explicit instruction on appropriate sexual behaviour is more crucial for people with autism due to difficulties recognizing red flags and interpreting thoughts, feelings and behaviors of others."[92]

It should be mentioned at this point that OB/GYN providers must be mindful to observe for any signs/symptoms that their ASD patients are victims of sexual abuse. For children (or adults) with autism, the signs of sexual abuse may manifest differently. In her article "Sexual Abuse of Children with Autism: Factors That Increase Risk and Interfere with Recognition of Abuse," Dr. Meredyth Goldberg Edelson of Williamette University notes the following:

"Children with autism sometimes display self-stimulatory behaviors, self-injurious behaviors, and stereotypic and repetitive behaviors (APA, 2004; Cunningham and Schreibman, 2008). Should a child (or adult) be sexually abused, their attempt to cope with or make sense out of that abuse may lead to an increase in the intensity and frequency of these behaviors or to the development of new behaviors that were not previously present."[93]

"ASD patients who are non-verbal exhibit more behavioral difficulties than those who have verbal communication abilities (Dominic, Davis, Lanihart, Tager-Flusberg, & Folstein. 2007). This may relate to the frustration caused by the inability of others to understand what the ASD individual is trying to communicate. For the ASD individual who wishes to disclose their abuse, behavioral reactions to sexual abuse may develop if others cannot understand their communication about the abuse, but these behaviors may be misinterpreted by others as merely a manifestation of autism. Therefore, the fact that the ASD individual was, or continues to be, sexually abused may be missed."[94]

Making Your ASD Patient Comfortable During Exams

Due to the stressful nature of pelvic exams, it is the duty of the health care provider to develop a protocol for his or her ASD patients. None of these steps necessitate accruing expenses, just good planning and thoughtfulness. In fact, quite surely the rest of your patients would appreciate the same details. Remember, these extra steps constitute accommodating a patient with a disability, just the same as having a ramp to enter the building. ASD is an "invisible" disability, necessitating accommodations that must be provided.

Ask the ASD patient if she does breast self-exams. Even if she says yes, have a chart readily available to show her the correct way to do the exam. Provide information for further assistance. Suggest that she watch an instructional video on YouTube https://www.youtube.com/watch?v=MQKOA6TOHRA

For those needing a mammogram, the procedure should be discussed in detail, including what it will feel like. It may be that the ASD patient simply cannot tolerate the tight squeezing of the machine, which is necessary for good imaging. Additionally, the mammogram technician should also be educated about autism and how to best deal with the ASD patient.

1. Schedule the ASD patient as the first or last patient of the day to minimize waiting time.

2. Provide a separate room that is only for ASD patients. It should have dim lighting, with incandescent bulbs only. It should be quiet, with minimal furniture, no other patients or family members, calming spa colors and textures, and perhaps a small waterfall, away from the other patients. No television. If there

is any music, it should be only very soft, soothing music. Paint colors for the walls should be earth tones.

3. Allow the ASD patient to have a tour of the office and exam room prior to the actual appointment. This is an excellent time to introduce yourself and answer any questions she may have. It's also a good time to provide her with resources to read or go online to familiarize herself with what the exam will entail. An excellent source to provide her with is a website from the Mayo Clinic http://www.mayoclinic.org/tests-procedures/pap-smear/multimedia/pap-test/img-20007025

4. For ASD patients interested in information about the various methods of birth control available, an excellent site that provides a comprehensive list of every type of birth control can be found at http://www.arhp.org/methodmatch/

5. Before the ASD patient gets on the exam table, discuss each step of the exam and what will be taking place, and how it will feel. Give her time to process the information you just provided. Ask her if she has any questions or needs to hear anything a second time. Remain calm and patient, and use a soft gentle tone of voice. Explain both the pelvic exam and the breast exam, indicating that it will be done in that order. Let her get changed into the exam gown, indicating to put it on so that it opens in the front. Explain that it needs to go on like that so you may perform the breast exam. Provide her with a warmed blanket with which she may cover herself after changing into the gown. This will be especially necessary for when she will be on the exam table with her feet in the stirrups and her legs apart. In particular, with the ASD patient who either has never had sexual relations or a patient who was sexually abused, getting into that position may be extremely emotionally traumatizing. Be patient, calm, and quiet, yet helpful. Ask direct questions regarding her stress. Hopefully she will be willing to share that with you. You may need to be creative, think outside the box, and be flexible in these situations.

6. Be sure the exam room is at a pleasant temperature. Provide disposable socks for her to put on in case she doesn't have socks on when she arrives. That will prevent coldness violation when her feet go in the stirrups. The exam room should also have a Bair Hugger machine with a warming blanket to cover the exam table so there isn't a shock when the ASD patient gets on the table. A warm blanket should be readily available to cover her from the waist down. Speculums should be kept in a warming device until ready to use. Extreme temperature changes are to be avoided as not to cause massive sensory overload.

7.   Lighting in the exam room should be subdued, using only incandescent bulbs instead of fluorescent lights, which cause sensory disturbances to most ASD individuals.

8.   Be sure there will be no disturbances during the exam, such as staff members knocking on the door or entering the room, no phones or pagers going off, and all necessary equipment is readily available and ready to go.

9.   Review one last time with the ASD patient the steps of the exam. Tell her you will state them as the actual exam is being done as well. Allow her time to think of any last-minute questions she might have.

10. Reassure her that you will be quick with the exam, will announce each step before its done, and no small talk will occur. ASD individuals do not like small talk, least of all done during a pelvic exam. Keep all communication direct and to the point. Remember to remain calm at all times, keep your voice soft, and maintain a professional expression on your face. Even if the ASD patient begins to have a meltdown, simply remain calm. Do not exhibit annoyance or any such emotion. Describe ahead of time what each step will feel like and where there will be discomfort.

11. Finally, have her get on the table. Proceed with the exam as already described. State each step before you do it. Be sure the speculum is warm prior to insertion. Be direct and narrate each step in as few words as possible. Once the pelvic exam is complete, let her cover herself. Proceed with the breast exam. Again, make no small talk. Just alert her of what you will be doing before you do it. Be sure your hands are warm before touching her breasts. Best point: after the pelvic exam, remove your gloves and wash your hands in very warm water. Then immediately proceed with the breast exam.

12. Once the exam is complete, the ASD patient may get up from the exam table and get dressed back into her clothing. Step out of the room to allow her to dress, just as is done with every patient. Once she is completed dressing, return to discuss the exam and any findings. Provide her with information regarding how she will receive her results. If there are choices, please offer them.

13. Remember to treat your ASD patient with the same respect and dignity as all your other patients. She has the same needs for love and relationships as others do. While there are some ASD individuals who are asexual, most are interested in sex and becoming sexually active or are already sexually active. Be pre-

pared to discuss questions they have with the same level of information as you'd give your other patients. Don't provide less information because you think they are "disabled" and don't require much information. Also, don't judge them by their facial expressions, which may be complete void. Additionally, don't expect much eye contact from your ASD patient.

14. Expect that you will need to spend more time with the ASD patient. If at any time during the exam the ASD patient indicates the desire to stop, do so immediately. Let her regroup, calm down, breathe slowly, or whatever she needs.

At the conclusion of the procedure, praise her for a job well done in going through a difficult exam. Acknowledge that you understand how difficult it was for her. Your kind words will go a long way. Remind her to do her monthly breast self-exam. Finish up by asking if she has any further questions.

Footnotes

90. http://link.springer.com/article/10.1007/s10803-014-2093-y/fulltext.html

91. https://www.autismspeaks.org/family-services/autism-safety-project/sexual-abuse

92. http://www.medicaldaily.com/sex-abuse-risk-higher-people-autism-prompting-calls-better-sex-education-298430

93. https://www.autismspeaks.org/family-services/autism-safety-project/sexual-abuse

94. https://www.autismspeaks.org/family-services/autism-safety-project/sexual-abuse

Chapter 18
HIPAA Requirements

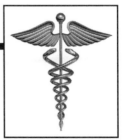

Health care providers are already familiar with HIPAA and the seriousness of its implications on everyday practice in the medical world. Regarding ASD patients, the same rules apply to this patient population just as all the rest. In order to be sure the laws and regulations are clearly understood, I felt it necessary to include it in its entirety. Of importance is the Privacy portion, as anyone violating this law can receive massive fines and be arrested on criminal penalties.

The Health Insurance Portability and Accountability Act of 1966 (HIPAA) was enacted by the United States Congress and signed by President Bill Clinton in 1996. It has been known as the Kennedy-Kassebaum Act after two of its leading sponsors. Title I of HIPAA protects health insurance coverage for workers and their families when they change or lose their jobs. Title II of HIPAA, known as the Administrative Simplification provisions, requires the establishment of national standards for electronic health care transactions and national identifiers for providers, health insurance plans, and employers. [95]

The most comprehensive version of HIPAA was found on Wikipedia. It is not intended for the reader to read the HIPAA Act below at the website, but to have it to refer to for specific regulations regarding patient privacy and what happens when those regulations are violated.

Footnotes

95.   https://en.wikipedia.org/wiki/Health_Insurance_Portability_and_Accountability_Act

Chapter 19

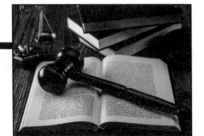

Americans with Disabilities Act

The Americans with Disabilities Act of 1990 is a United States labor law that prohibits unjustified discrimination based on disability. It affords similar protections against discrimination to Americans with disabilities as the **Civil Rights Act of 1964**, which made discrimination based on race, religion, sex, national origin, and other characteristics illegal. In addition, unlike the Civil Rights Act, the ADA also requires covered employers to provide reasonable accommodations to employees with disabilities and impose accessibility requirements on public accommodations.[97]

In 1986, the National Council on Disability had recommended enactment of an Americans with Disabilities Act (ADA) and drafted the first version of the bill, which was introduced in the House and Senate in 1988. The final version of the bill was signed into law on July 26, 1990 by President George H.W. Bush. It was later amended in 2008 and signed by President George W. Bush with changes effective as of January 1, 2009.[98]

As with HIPAA, the Americans with Disabilities Act isn't intended to be read through in its entirety. It is included for using as your reference concerning those with disabilities.

U.S. Department of Justice
Civil Rights Division | Disability Rights Section

Title III Highlights

I.   Who is covered by title III of the ADA

II. Overview of Requirements

III. Individuals with Disabilities

IV. Eligibility for Goods and Services

V.   Modifications in Policies, Practices, and Procedures

VI. Auxiliary Aids

VII. Existing Facilities: Removal of Barriers

VIII. Existing Facilities: Alternatives to Barrier Removal

IX. New Construction

X.   Alterations

XI. Overview of Americans with Disabilities Act Accessibility Guidelines for New Construction and Alterations

XII. Examinations and Courses

XIII. Enforcement of the ADA and its Regulations

XIV. Technical Assistance

I. Who is Covered by Title III of the ADA

The title III regulation covers:

- Public accommodations (i.e., private entities that own, operate, lease, or lease to places of public accommodation),

- Commercial facilities, and

- Private entities that offer certain examinations and courses related to educational and occupational certification.

Chapter 19: Americans with Disabilities Act

- Places of public accommodation include over five million private establishments, such as restaurants, hotels, theaters, convention centers, retail stores, shopping centers, dry cleaners, laundromats, pharmacies, doctors' offices, hospitals, museums, libraries, parks, zoos, amusement parks, private schools, day care centers, health spas, and bowling alleys.

- Commercial facilities are nonresidential facilities, including office buildings, factories, and warehouses, whose operations affect commerce.

- Entities controlled by religious organizations, including places of worship, are not covered.

- Private clubs are not covered, except to the extent that the facilities of the private club are made available to customers or patrons of a place of public accommodation.

- State and local governments are not covered by the title III regulation, but rather by the Department of Justice's title II regulation.

II. Overview of Requirements

Public accommodations must:

- Provide goods and services in an integrated setting, unless separate or different measures are necessary to ensure equal opportunity.

- Eliminate unnecessary eligibility standards or rules that deny individuals with disabilities an equal opportunity to enjoy the goods and services of a place of public accommodation.

- Make reasonable modifications in policies, practices, and procedures that deny equal access to individuals with disabilities, unless a fundamental alteration would result in the nature of the goods and services provided.

- Furnish auxiliary aids when necessary to ensure effective communication, unless an undue burden or fundamental alteration would result.

- Remove architectural and structural communication barriers in existing facilities where readily achievable.

- Provide readily achievable alternative measures when removal of barriers is not readily achievable.

- Provide equivalent transportation services and purchase accessible vehicles in certain circumstances.

- Maintain accessible features of facilities and equipment.

- Design and construct new facilities and, when undertaking alterations, alter existing facilities in accordance with the Americans with Disabilities Act Accessibility Guidelines issued by the Architectural and Transportation Barriers Compliance Board and incorporated in the final Department of Justice title III regulation.

- A public accommodation is not required to provide personal devices such as wheelchairs; individually prescribed devices (e.g., prescription eyeglasses or hearing aids); or services of a personal nature including assistance in eating, toileting, or dressing.

- A public accommodation may not discriminate against an individual or entity because of the known disability of a person with whom the individual or entity is known to associate.

- Commercial facilities are only subject to the requirement that new construction and alterations conform to the ADA Accessibility Guidelines. The other requirements applicable to public accommodations listed above do not apply to commercial facilities.

- Private entities offering certain examinations or courses (i.e., those related to applications, licensing, certification, or credentialing for secondary or postsecondary education, professional, or trade purposes) must offer them in an accessible place and manner or offer alternative accessible arrangements.

III. *"Individuals with Disabilities"*

The Americans with Disabilities Act provides comprehensive civil rights protections for "individuals with disabilities."

An individual with a disability is a person who:

- Has a physical or mental impairment that substantially limits one or more major life activities, or

- Has a record of such an impairment, or

- Is regarded as having such an impairment.

- Examples of physical or mental impairments include, but are not limited to, such contagious and non-contagious diseases and conditions as orthopedic, visual, speech, and hearing impairments; cerebral palsy, epilepsy, muscular dystrophy, multiple sclerosis, cancer, heart disease, diabetes, mental retardation, emotional illness, specific learning disabilities, HIV disease (whether symptomatic or asymptomatic), tuberculosis, drug addiction, and alcoholism. Homosexuality and bisexuality are not physical or mental impairments under the ADA.

- "Major life activities" include functions such as caring for oneself, performing manual tasks, walking, seeing, hearing, speaking, breathing, learning, and working.

- Individuals who currently engage in the illegal use of drugs are not protected by the ADA when an action is taken on the basis of their current illegal use of drugs.

IV. Eligibility for Goods and Services

- In providing goods and services, a public accommodation may not use eligibility requirements that exclude or segregate individuals with disabilities, unless the requirements are *necessary* for the operation of the public accommodation.

   For example, excluding individuals with cerebral palsy from a movie theater or restricting individuals with Down's Syndrome to only certain areas of a restaurant would violate the regulation.

- Requirements that tend to screen out individuals with disabilities, such as requiring a blind person to produce a driver's license as the sole means of identification for cashing a check, are also prohibited.

- Safety requirements may be imposed only if they are necessary for the safe operation of a place of public accommodation. They must be based on actual risks and not on mere speculation, stereotypes, or generalizations about individuals with disabilities.

   For example, an amusement park may impose height requirements for certain rides when required for safety.

- Extra charges may not be imposed on individuals with disabilities to cover the costs of measures necessary to ensure nondiscriminatory treatment, such as removing barriers or providing qualified interpreters.

V. Modifications in Policies, Practices, and Procedures

- A public accommodation must make reasonable modifications in its policies, practices, and procedures in order to accommodate individuals with disabilities.

- A modification is not required if it would "fundamentally alter" the goods, services, or operations of the public accommodation.

- For example, a department store may need to modify a policy of only permitting one person at a time in a dressing room if an individual with mental retardation needs the assistance of a companion in dressing.

- Modifications in existing practices generally must be made to permit the use of guide dogs and other service animals.

- Specialists are not required to provide services outside of their legitimate areas of specialization.

- For example, a doctor who specializes exclusively in burn treatment may refer an individual with a disability, who is not seeking burn treatment, to another provider. A burn specialist, however, could not refuse to provide burn treatment to, for example, an individual with HIV disease.

VI. *Auxiliary Aids*

- A public accommodation must provide auxiliary aids and services when they are necessary to ensure effective communication with individuals with hearing, vision, or speech impairments.

- "Auxiliary aids" include such services or devices as qualified interpreters, assistive listening headsets, television captioning and decoders, telecommunications devices for deaf persons (TDD's), videotext displays, readers, taped texts, Braille materials, and large-print materials.

- The auxiliary aid requirement is flexible. For example, a Braille menu is not required, if waiters are instructed to read the menu to blind customers.

- Auxiliary aids that would result in an undue burden, (i.e., "significant difficulty or expense") or in a fundamental alteration in the nature of the goods or services are not required by the regulation. However, a public accommodation must still furnish another auxiliary aid, if available, that does not result in a fundamental alteration or an undue burden.

VII. *Existing Facilities: Removal of Barriers*

- Physical barriers to entering and using existing facilities must be removed when "readily achievable."

- Readily achievable means "easily accomplishable and able to be carried out without much difficulty or expense."

- What is readily achievable will be determined on a case-by-case basis in light of the resources available.

- The regulation does not require the rearrangement of temporary or movable structures, such as furniture, equipment, and display racks to the extent that it would result in a significant loss of selling or serving space.

- Legitimate safety requirements may be considered in determining what is readily achievable so long as they are based on actual risks and are necessary for safe operation.

- Examples of barrier removal measures include --
  - Installing ramps,
  - Making curb cuts at sidewalks and entrances,
  - Rearranging tables, chairs, vending machines, display racks, and other furniture,
  - Widening doorways,
  - Installing grab bars in toilet stalls, and
  - Adding raised letters or braille to elevator control buttons.

- First priority should be given to measures that will enable individuals with disabilities to "get in the front door," followed by measures to provide access to areas providing goods and services.

- Barrier removal measures must comply, when readily achievable, with the alterations requirements of the ADA Accessibility Guidelines. If compliance with the Guidelines is not readily achievable, other safe, readily achievable measures must be taken, such as installation of a slightly narrower door than would be required by the Guidelines.

VIII. Existing Facilities: Alternatives to Barrier Removal

- The ADA requires the removal of physical barriers, such as stairs, if it is "readily achievable." However, if removal is not readily achievable, alternative steps must be taken to make goods and services accessible.

- Examples of alternative measures include --
  - Providing goods and services at the door, sidewalk, or curb,
  - Providing home delivery,
  - Retrieving merchandise from inaccessible shelves or racks,
  - Relocating activities to accessible locations.

- Extra charges may not be imposed on individuals with disabilities to cover the costs of measures used as alternatives to barrier removal. For example, a restaurant may not charge a wheelchair user extra for home delivery when it is provided as the alternative to barrier removal.

IX. New Construction

- All newly constructed places of public accommodation and commercial facilities must be accessible to individuals with disabilities to the extent that it is not structurally impracticable.
- The new construction requirements apply to any facility occupied after January 26, 1993, for which the last application for a building permit or permit extension is certified as complete after January 26, 1992.
- Full compliance will be considered "structurally impracticable" only in those rare circumstances when the unique characteristics of terrain prevent the incorporation of accessibility features (e.g., marshland that requires construction on stilts).
- The architectural standards for accessibility in new construction are contained in the ADA Accessibility Guidelines issued by the Architectural and Transportation Barriers Compliance Board, an independent Federal agency. These standards are incorporated in the final Department of Justice title III regulation.
- Elevators are not required in facilities under three stories or with fewer than 3,000 square feet per floor, unless the building is a shopping center, shopping mall, professional office of a health care provider, or station used for public transportation.

X. Alterations

- Alterations after January 26, 1992, to existing places of public accommodation and commercial facilities must be accessible to the maximum extent feasible.
- The architectural standards for accessibility in alterations are contained in the ADA Accessibility Guidelines issued by the Architectural and Transportation Barriers Compliance Board. These standards are incorporated in the final Department of Justice title III regulation.
- An alteration is a change that affects usability of a facility. For example, if during remodeling, renovation, or restoration, a doorway is being relocated, the new doorway must be wide enough to meet the requirements of the ADA Accessibility Guidelines.

Chapter 19: Americans with Disabilities Act

- When alterations are made to a "primary function area", such as the lobby or work areas of a bank, an accessible path of travel to the altered area, and the bathrooms, telephones, and drinking fountains serving that area, must be made accessible to the extent that the added accessibility costs are not disproportionate to the overall cost of the original alteration.

- Alterations to windows, hardware, controls, electrical outlets, and signage in primary function areas do not trigger the path of travel requirement.

- The added accessibility costs are disproportionate if they exceed 20 percent of the original alteration.

- Elevators are not required in facilities under three stories or with fewer than 3,000 square feet per floor, unless the building is a shopping center, shopping mall, professional office of a health care provider, or station used for public transportation.

XI. Overview of Americans with Disabilities Act Accessibility Guidelines for New Construction and Alterations

- New construction and alterations must be accessible in compliance with the ADA Accessibility Guidelines.

- The Guidelines contain general design ("technical") standards for building and site elements, such as parking, accessible routes, ramps, stairs, elevators, doors, entrances, drinking fountains, bathrooms, controls and operating mechanisms, storage areas, alarms, signage, telephones, fixed seating and tables, assembly areas, automated teller machines, and dressing rooms. They also have specific technical standards for restaurants, medical care facilities, mercantile facilities, libraries, and transient lodging (such as hotels and shelters).

- The Guidelines also contain "scoping" requirements for various elements (i.e., it specifies how many, and under what circumstances, accessibility features must be incorporated).

- Following are examples of scoping requirements in new construction:
  - At least 50 percent of all public entrances must be accessible. In addition, there must be accessible entrances to enclosed parking, pedestrian tunnels, and elevated walkways.
  - An accessible route must connect accessible public transportation stops, parking spaces, passenger loading zones, and public streets or sidewalks to all accessible features and spaces within a building.

- Every public and common use bathroom must be accessible. Only one stall must be accessible, unless there are six or more stalls, in which case two stalls must be accessible (one of which must be of an alternate, narrow-style design).

- Each floor in a building without a supervised sprinkler system must contain an "area of rescue assistance" (i.e., an area with direct access to an exit stairway where people unable to use stairs may await assistance during an emergency evacuation).

- One TDD must be provided inside any building that has four or more public pay telephones, counting both interior and exterior phones. In addition, one TDD must be provided whenever there is an interior public pay phone in a stadium or arena; convention center; hotel with a convention center; covered shopping mall; or hospital emergency, recovery, or waiting room.

- One accessible public phone must be provided for each floor, unless the floor has two or more banks of phones, in which case there must be one accessible phone for each bank.

- Fixed seating assembly areas that accommodate 50 or more people or have audio-amplification systems must have a permanently installed assistive listening system.

- Dispersal of wheelchair seating in theaters is required where there are more than 300 seats. In addition, at least one percent of all fixed seats must be aisle seats without armrests (or with movable armrests). Fixed seating for companions must be located adjacent to each wheelchair location.

- Where automated teller machines are provided, at least one must be accessible.

- Five percent of fitting and dressing rooms (but never less than one) must be accessible.

- Following are examples of specific scoping requirements for new construction of special types of facilities, such as restaurants, medical care facilities, mercantile establishments, libraries, and hotels:

  - In restaurants, generally all dining areas and five percent of fixed tables (but not less than one) must be accessible.

  - In medical care facilities, all public and common use areas must be accessible. In general purpose hospitals and in psychiatric and detoxification facilities, ten percent of patient bedrooms and toilets must be accessible. The required percentage is 100 percent for special facilities treating conditions that affect mobility, and 50 percent for long-term care facilities and nursing homes.

- In mercantile establishments, at least one of each type of counter containing a cash register and at least one of each design of check-out aisle must be accessible. In some cases, additional check-out aisles are required to be accessible (i.e., from 20 to 40 percent) depending on the number of check-out aisles and the size of the facility.

- In libraries, all public areas must be accessible. In addition, five percent of fixed tables or study carrels (or at least one) must be accessible. At least one lane at the check-out area and aisles between card catalogs, magazine displays, and stacks must be accessible.

- In hotels, four percent of the first 100 rooms and approximately two percent of rooms in excess of 100 must be accessible to persons with hearing impairments (i.e., contain visual alarms, visual notification devices, volume-control telephones, and an accessible electrical outlet for a TDD) and to persons with mobility impairments. Moreover, an identical percentage of additional rooms must be accessible to persons with hearing impairments.

- Technical and scoping requirements for alterations are sometimes less stringent than those for new construction. For example, when compliance with the new construction requirements would be technically infeasible, one accessible unisex bathroom per floor is acceptable.

XII. Examinations and Courses

Certain examinations or courses offered by a private entity (i.e., those that are related to applications, licensing, certification, or credentialing for secondary or postsecondary education, professional, or trade purposes) must either be given in a place and manner accessible to persons with disabilities, or be made accessible through alternative means.

In order to provide an examination in an accessible place and manner, a private entity must:

- Assure that the examination measures what it is intended to measure, rather than reflecting the individual's impaired sensory, manual, or speaking skills.

- Modify the examination format when necessary (e.g., permit additional time).

- Provide auxiliary aids (e.g., taped exams, interpreters, large print answer sheets, or qualified readers), unless they would fundamentally alter the measurement of the skills or knowledge that the examination is intended to test or would result in an undue burden.

- Offer any modified examination at an equally convenient location, as often, and in as timely a manner as are other examinations.

- Administer examinations in a facility that is accessible or provide alternative comparable arrangements, such as providing the examination at an individual's home with a proctor.

- In order to provide a course in an accessible place and manner, a private entity may need to:

  - Modify the course format or requirements (e.g., permit additional time for completion of the course).

  - Provide auxiliary aids, unless a fundamental alteration or undue burden would result.

  - Administer the course in a facility that is accessible or provide alternative comparable arrangements, such as provision of the course through video tape, audio cassettes, or prepared notes.

XIII. Enforcement of the ADA and its Regulations

- Private parties may bring lawsuits to obtain court orders to stop discrimination. No monetary damages will be available in such suits. A reasonable attorney's fee, however, may be awarded.

- Individuals may also file complaints with the Attorney General who is authorized to bring lawsuits in cases of general public importance or where a "pattern or practice" of discrimination is alleged.

- In suits brought by the Attorney General, monetary damages (not including punitive damages) and civil penalties may be awarded. Civil penalties may not exceed $50,000 for a first violation or $100,000 for any subsequent violation.

XIV. Technical Assistance

- The ADA requires that the Federal agencies responsible for issuing ADA regulations provide "technical assistance."

- Technical assistance is the dissemination of information (either directly by the Department or through grants and contracts) to assist the public, including individuals protected by the ADA and entities covered by the ADA, in understanding the new law.

- Methods of providing information include, for example, audio-visual materials, pamphlets, manuals, electronic bulletin boards, checklists, and training.

- The Department issued for public comment on December 5, 1990, a government-wide plan for the provision of technical assistance.

- The Department's efforts focus on raising public awareness of the ADA by providing:

  - Fact sheets and pamphlets in accessible formats,

  - Speakers for workshops, seminars, classes, and conferences,

  - An ADA telephone information line, and

  - Access to ADA documents through an electronic bulletin board for users of personal computers.

- The Department has established a comprehensive program of technical assistance relating to public accommodations and State and local governments.

- Grants will be awarded for projects to inform individuals with disabilities and covered entities about their rights and responsibilities under the ADA and to facilitate voluntary compliance.

- The Department will issue a technical assistance manual by January 26, 1992, for individuals or entities with rights or duties under the ADA.

For additional information, contact:

Disability Rights Section

Civil Rights Division

U.S. Department of Justice

P.O. Box 66738

Washington, D.C 20035-6738

(800) 514-0301 (Voice)

(800) 514-0383 (TDD)

(202) 514-6193 (Electronic Bulletin Board)

The Americans with Disabilities Act primarily focuses on providing accommodations for people with mobility disabilities. It is understandable that health care providers may not be aware that autism is included in the ADA and that this population requires special accommodations as well. Obviously, everywhere you go today, there are ramps, elevators, wider entryways, restrooms with necessary accommodations, etc. That is all necessary for those with the physical handicaps.

But where are the accommodations for those with autism? As you have already learned from previous chapters, autistic individuals have many sensory issues. Things that have a significant effect on them include lighting, sounds, the frequency of sounds, textures, color, movement, temperature, tone of voice of others, and facial expressions. When an ASD patient first walks through the door into a health care facility, the environment they are confronted with will greatly affect them, for better or for worse.

In order to promote a successful outcome at the conclusion of their visit, accommodations must be addressed just like those for the physically disabled. Many of the accommodations necessary for ASD patients can be done at little or no cost. However, some health care facilities are investing money into creating even more enticing autism-friendly accommodations. Waiting areas with a waterfall or large tropical fish tank, indirect soft lighting, slate flooring, soft-textured chairs and couches, lots of live plants, and soft soothing music act to calm the ASD patient. At the reception desk, many places are now having the reception team behind a glass window, which has a sliding window to speak with patients as they check in. The rest of the time the window is kept closed, which greatly limits the noise of phones ringing and staff talking heard in the waiting area. In fact, the other non-autistic patients will surely enjoy the spa-like ambiance of an ASD environment.

Within any community, word will spread quickly through the autistic population that a health care facility is autism friendly. Remember, the environment is only the beginning. Knowledge of autism and how to effectively communicate with this unique group of individuals is the key to successful health care for them.

Footnotes

97.   https://en.wikipedia.org/wiki/Americans_with_Disabilities_Act_of_1990

98.   https://en.wikipedia.org/wiki/Americans_with_Disabilities_Act_of_1990

Chapter 20
Putting All the
Pieces Together

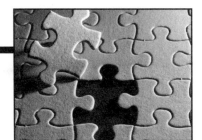

Just like the pieces of the autism puzzle, this book has given you many pieces to assemble into the finished picture. By now you should have a solid foundation on which to build your care of ASD patients.

Case Scenario

Six-year-old Sergei was recently diagnosed with autism. His parents are still in the denial stage of his diagnosis. His neurologist has put in a referral for an MRI under general anesthesia. It is scheduled at a local hospital. There are several hospitals in the area, but the neurologist selects the one at which all staff have been in-serviced on autism with The Complete Guide to Autism for Health Care Professionals & Ancillary Staff. From the secretary at the admissions desk through the checkout clerk at the discharge area, everyone understands what autism is AND the best ways to deal with ASD patients.

A nurse from the hospital's MRI department calla Sergei's mom a week ahead of the scheduled MRI. She informs Sergei's mom, Mary, that the hospital is autism-friendly, and she needs to gather information prior to the day of the MRI. Mary is very relieved that the nurse has called and that her son will receive special attention. The nurse proceeds with asking the questions on the Autism Care Questionnaire. After the whole form has been completed, the nurse asks Mary if she has any questions. The nurse informs Mary that, upon arrival to the hospital, once she checks in at the admissions desk, she and Sergei will be transported to their autism waiting room. Mary is very pleased, commenting that she was fearful of having to wait a long time in a busy waiting area, worried that Sergei would have a meltdown. The nurse asks Mary if Sergei has a favorite blanket, cup, or toy. Mary replies that he has a teddy bear, a blanket, and a plastic cup that he loves. The nurse tells Mary to bring all three items on the day of his MRI. The call is concluded with final instructions from the nurse, which includes telling Mary to go online to the hospital's website to look at the videos of getting an MRI.

Two things have now occurred: 1) The nurse has gathered all necessary information to understand Sergei, how he communicates, what his stress triggers are, how to recognize when a meltdown might be coming, what comforts him, and any past experiences with other procedures. This information will be passed along to all who will be caring for Sergei. The second thing that occurred is that Mary's anxiety level has dramatically decreased, knowing that she is bringing Sergei to a facility where they understand autism and will be ready to deal with Sergei. Mary feels like she can trust they will do the right thing with her precious little boy. To a parent of a child with ASD, this is a gift.

The nurse who spoke with Mary will record all the information in the chart she is preparing for Sergei, of course maintaining complete confidentiality in compliance with HIPAA regulations. She then meets with the staff member who will be taking care of Sergei on the day he comes for his MRI. This will include the pre-op area, the MRI staff, and the Post Anesthesia Care Unit (PACU), and the discharge staff. She will also alert the admissions staff as well. In the chart, the nurse will include the release form that the hospital has developed for the parent/caregiver/patient to sign, giving permission to get the Autism ID bracelet. Once the bracelet is on the patient, it will alert all staff to employ the autism protocol. This maintains the continuity of care in the event that one or more of the staff was not available when the information was passed along.

At home, Mary begins preparation for the big day. She has one week to get Sergei ready. First, Mary gets on her computer and goes to the hospital's website. She quickly locates the ASD area and sees "Your Child with ASD is getting an MRI." First she watches the video herself. She is very pleased to see that it shows every step of the way from the moment she will arrive at the hospital through the pre-op area, a patient getting ready with a nurse helping, and all the medical devices that Sergei will be seeing and what will be done to him. The staff in the video is the actual staff that will be caring for him.

Chapter 20: Putting All the Pieces Together

After watching the entire video, Mary brings Sergei over to watch it with her. She explains to him that he needs to have a special picture taken of his head. She tells him they will be going to the hospital the following week and he will be seeing new people. She also tells him she wants him to watch the video so he can see what will occur when he is there. As Sergei watches, he sees that the little boy in the video looks very happy and seems to be having fun. Mary continues to sit with him as he watches. Sergei wants to see it again, so they end up watching it four more times. Sergei seems very interested that he will get to go there and have fun like the little boy in the video. Mary then asks him to help her pack the bag they will take to the hospital. This makes Sergei feel very important that he is getting to help pack. He wants to bring his soft fuzzy microfleece blanket, his good friend "Huggy," the well-worn teddy bear, and a plastic cup that he drinks out of for everything. Mary has the bag ready to go.

Over the next few days, Mary has Sergei watch the video numerous times. Two days before the appointment, Mary tells Sergei they are going for a ride to see the hospital. Sergei has never been there before or been on that route. Along the way, Mary tells him to look at restaurants along the way, and pick out one of them he'd like to go to on the way home after his day at the hospital. Sergei loves milkshakes, and there happens to be a burger place that makes great milkshakes along the route. Sergei is very excited that he will be getting a milkshake after his special picture of his head is all done.

Once at the hospital, Mary takes Sergei in to see where he will be going in two more days. They go to the admissions desk, then to the pre-op area where he'll be prepared for his MRI. The nurse who had initially spoken with Mary is there in the pre-op area. She greets them with a soft, calm voice. Sergei recognizes the area from the video he watched. The nurse shows him the area he will be in to get ready for the MRI. It looks just like the video. Two of the staff from the MRI area come out to greet Sergei. He looks down at the floor, but they continue talking to him in the same calm, soft voice as the nurse. They simply say hello to him by name and assure him that they will be with him in two days. They don't attempt to touch Sergei or talk excessively. The Certified Registered Nurse Anesthetist who will be giving his anesthesia also comes to see Sergei. She introduces herself and tells Sergei that she will be helping with his special picture as well. He looks up at them as he is leaving, and they wave good-bye to him. Sergei waves back at them.

On the way home, Sergei wants to get a milkshake, but Mary tells him he has to wait until after his special pictures are done in two days, and on the way home from that he can get one. Once home, Mary shows him the video again. Now he is excited because he has seen the people in person. He now feels comfortable about going for his MRI. Mary also tells Sergei that they can't eat breakfast on the morning of the special pictures. Sergei isn't very happy about that, but Mary explains that it's very important that he has an empty stomach because he must have a nap while the pictures are being taken.

Finally the big day arrives. On the way out the door of the house, Sergei wants to carry the bag with all his favorite things. On the way to the hospital, Mary reminds him of the great milkshake he's going to get later. Sergei states he wants a vanilla shake, and Mary is pleased that he's now focused on his treat!

They walk into the hospital and proceed to the admissions desk. Once signed in, a transport person arrives and takes them to the special autism waiting room. Mary was given the release form to sign to allow the autism bracelet to be placed on Sergei's wrist. First the admission's clerk shows it to him, shows how it goes on by pretending to put it on Mary's wrist, then Sergei allows her to place it on his wrist. When the transport person has arrived, they see the autism wristband and know how to enact the autism protocol. It's dimly lit and quiet. No one else is in the room except Mary and Sergei. It is very calming, especially with the waterfall in the corner with many plants by it. Sergei walks over to watch the water. He is very interested in it. He's even more interested when he spots an area with some fun things to do. Looking in a big box, he sees small boxes of crayons, several coloring books, and a variety of squishy toys. Mary tells him he may choose something to do from the box. Sergei loves to color, so he gets a box of crayons and a coloring book. He brings his new items by Mary and begins to color. He's just gotten underway, and a nurse comes in to take them to the MRI pre-op area. Sergei has the first appointment of the day, so they haven't waited long before being taken into the next area.

In the pre-op area, a nurse that Sergei recognizes from the video comes to greet them. He is in the special pre-op room used for ASD patients. It is dimly lit, away from the other patients, with a chair for Mary and the stretcher. The nurse introduces herself, then gives Sergei a gown to change into. Sergei also recognizes the gown from the video, the same one the little boy had on! After he is changed, the nurse returns. She shows him the blood pressure cuff and puts it on Mary to show him how it looks. He puts his arm out, and the nurse puts on the cuff. She then shows him the pulse oximeter, again placing it on Mary first. Sergei is excited to see the red light coming from the pulse oximeter. Last comes the little sticky EKG patches. The nurse first shows him the stickers, then points where she is going to place them on him. Sergei is familiar with these monitors because he saw the procedure multiple times on the video. He feels brave, just like the little boy was.

Sergei then climbs up on the stretcher. Once there, the nurse anesthetist/anesthesiologist comes to see him. She brings along the mask that will be used in the MRI room. Sergei takes the mask and plays with it, holding it on his face like he saw the little boy do in the video. It is already planned to do an inhalation induction and place the IV once he is asleep. So far, everything is going very smoothly. Sergei is not exhibiting any signs of stress or fear. Mary is right there, and he has his teddy bear and cozy blanket. It is decided that, in order to keep things going smoothly, that Sergei would get some Versed to drink. Using his favorite cup, the nurse mixes up the drink of Versed 0.25 mg/kg with a tiny amount of apple juice. The anesthesia will consist simply of oxygen with inhalation anesthetic. No nitrous oxide will be used. Once he is asleep, an IV will be secured and normal saline given. The plan is to hydrate Sergei well so that no other drugs will need to be given to him. The fluid administration will prevent the need for antiemetics. Sergei is excited to get his special drink.

They wait 30 minutes before heading back to the MRI room. Meanwhile, as Sergei rests on his stretcher with his favorite blanket covering him, hugging teddy, the nurse anesthetist is busy preparing the MRI scanner room. The lights are dimmed down, the staff reviews what to do and what not to do, the radio is shut off, and the room temperature is set at 72 degrees.

Finally, it is time to bring Sergei to the MRI room. Mary is allowed to accompany him right into the scanner room. Sergei still has his mask, and the nurse anesthetist/anesthesiologist places it back on the breathing circuit of the anesthesia machine. Other than holding the mask over his face, Sergei doesn't need any other touching. His monitors are already in place from the pre-op area, which the nurse anesthetist simply reconnects the cables into her monitor. Mary is allowed to stay there until he drifts off to sleep. At that point, Mary and the pre-op nurse who has also come along, leave the room. Now under general anesthesia, an IV is started in his hand and lightly wrapped with web roll. Sergei is then lifted onto the MRI scanner bed and the MRI completed. The people who lifted him have stayed out of sight until he is safely asleep.

After the MRI, Sergei is transferred back onto his stretcher, covered with his blanket, teddy under his arm, and extubated when safe to do so. No one talks during this time except the nurse anesthetist/anesthesiologist as necessary. No one touches him except for what's medically necessary. There is no music playing, and no one makes any kind of noise in the room. He is then slowly transported to the recovery area and wheeled into one of the rooms designated for the ASD patients. The room is dimly lit quiet, and Mary is already in there awaiting him to arrive. The monitor cables are attached to the monitor in the room, so there is no need to be touching him to place the monitors on him. As he wakes up, he feels his soft blanket against his skin, he sees Mary right there, and its simply peaceful and quiet.

When it's time for discharge, the clerk comes to the room Sergei and Mary are in and has Mary sign all the discharge papers. The recovery room nurse reviews all the post-anesthesia care orders with Mary. Once all that is complete, a transport person arrives with a wheel chair. Sergei is ready to head on home, but not before he gets his treat! The recovery room nurse accompanies them out to the area where they bring Mary's car. They help Sergei into the vehicle, and now it's time to head home. Sergei has his crayons and coloring book, and is saying "milk-shake" over and over. When Mary pulls into the parking lot of the burger place, Sergei is very happy. She gets him his shake to drink now and one to take home.

Once home, it's time for a nap for both of them. With this scenario, it can clearly be seen the coordinated effort of the staff involved. It is apparent the limited number of people who encountered Sergei. There was no music or TV playing anywhere near him. Despite Sergei being absolutely adorable, with his thick blond hair and crystal-blue eyes, no one touched him or talked about it. He didn't have a meltdown because sensory stimuli was kept to a bare minimum. Also, because he had seen the video multiple times, he already felt comfortable and felt like he was in a familiar place.

Chapter 21
Parents: The
Unsung Heroes

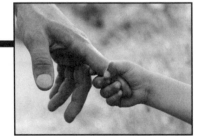

Every parent wants to have a perfectly normal baby handed to them in the delivery room. An expectant mother goes through nine months of pregnancy, labor, and delivery. During that time, she's dreaming of her new little boy or girl, imagining doing all the "normal" things with their child, watching him playing, having fun, and growing up. She might even be thinking far ahead, envisioning her baby as an adult, getting married and giving her a grandchild. Sadly, life doesn't always work out as planned. I have heard many parents describe the day they received their child's autism diagnosis. Mostly they describe a feeling that their life is over. They feel scared, lost, depressed, and even grief. They often are in denial for some time. I've heard some describe it as feeling like a family member passed away; the intensity is that deep.

Most parents then become very strong advocates for their autistic child. They do endless research and join countless online autism organizations. Their entire life revolves around that child in the hopes of enabling that little boy or girl to grow up and have some semblance of a normal, happy, productive life. Because these parents are used to advocating for their child, they will continue to do so at your health care facility. Embrace this fact and realize that their input in their child's care will make your life easier!

Be mindful to offer support to the ASD patient's parent/caregiver whenever possible. You only will see him/her for a brief period of time. Remember that such parents are working tirelessly to help their child. A kind word, a hand gently placed on their shoulder, an offer of a hot beverage, and keeping them updated all goes a very long way.

I came across a wonderful piece by Steven Muller, from *The Homestead, Innovative Solutions for Autism*. The following is a list created by a mom of an autistic son, which was distributed by New York Collaborates for Autism. It is 11 things you should never say to parents of an autistic child, and 11 you should. This list was created by Karen Siff Exkorn, author of *The Autism Sourcebook: Everything You Need to Know about Diagnosis, Treatment, Coping and Healing—From a Mother Whose Child Recovered*.

1. Don't say: "Is your child a musical or artistic genius? What special gifts does he/she have?" Most individuals on the autism spectrum don't have any special gifts. Only about 10% have savant qualities.

    Instead, say, "How is your child doing?"

2. Don't say, "You'd never know by looking at her/him that she/he has autism! She/he looks so normal!" While the person speaking will think they are giving the parent a compliment, most parents won't take it as a compliment.

    Instead, say, "Your child is adorable!"

3. Don't say, "God doesn't give you what you can't handle" or "Everything happens for the best!" Unless you're the parent of a child on the spectrum, you don't really know just how much there is to handle. This statement minimizes the struggle they are going through. Despite the fact that you are trying to put a positive note on the situation, the parent will not feel that the diagnosis is the best. Over time, parents come to acceptance, and some come to view the diagnosis as a gift or give them a new perspective on life. But you aren't the one to tell them to reach those terms.

    Instead, say, "Is there anything I can do to help you out?" or "I'm here if you need to talk."

4. Don't say, "I know exactly what you're going through. My cousin has a friend whose neighbor's sister has a child with autism." You have no idea what that parent is going through.

    Instead, say, "I don't know what you are going through but willing to listen if you'd like to talk."

5. Don't say, "Do you have other children, and are they autistic too?"

    Instead, say, "Do you have other children?"

6. Don't say, "Why don't you try that new diet I saw on TV or a great treatment they just had in the newspaper!"

    Instead, say, "I've been doing some research on autism, and if you'd like, I can share it with you."

7. Don't say, "Don't you think you've put him/her through enough treatment? Just let him grow out of it." Or "Just accept him/her as he/she is. Why use treatment to try and change them?" Children do not spontaneously grow out of autism. Parents do accept their children for who they are, but like parents of typical children, they want to give their children every opportunity they can. This frequently translates into intensive treatments. Research shows the importance of early intervention, and treatment/support continues over the lifetime of the ASD individual.

    Instead, say, "What kind of treatment program are you using for your child?" or "What school does your child attend?"

8. Don't say, "It's such a burden to have to drive my kids to soccer practice and ballet classes every day!" Or "My kids are talking so much they are driving me crazy!" Please don't complain about all of the "normal" things that bother you as the parent of a typical child, at least not in front of a parent with a child on the autism spectrum. Most parents of children with autism dream of driving their kids to soccer or ballet, and parents of the 25% of nonverbal children on the spectrum dream about their children speaking one day. Be aware of and sensitive to their needs.

    Instead say, "Can I offer to drive your child to speech therapy or physical therapy?"

9. Don't say, "You should really make time for yourself. You need to relax. Maybe schedule a massage!" Life can be incredibly overwhelming, especially in the months following an autism diagnosis. Usually a parent wants to learn everything they can about autism. Taking time for them to relax isn't realistic.

    Instead, say, "If you ever feel like you need to take some time for yourself, I'd be happy to help out."

10. Don't say, "How's the marriage going? I hear the divorce rate is 80% among parents of kids with autism!" Many people seem to like to quote this statistic. It's false. Despite the additional stress of raising a child with autism, the statistics are similar to marriages with or without a child with autism.

    Instead, say, "Can I offer to babysit so you and your spouse can go out to dinner?"

11.   Don't say, "What caused your child's autism?" There's no known cause for autism. Hundreds of millions of dollars are being spent researching a cause. Theories about the cause of autism include heredity, genetics, and environmental factors.

Instead: Say nothing.[99]

Remember, these parents are advocating for their children with autism, getting them all the therapy and services they need to become the best that child possibly can be. A warm smile and kind gesture will make their day.

Footnotes

99.   http://www.thehomestead.org/saynot-say-parent-child-autism/

Chapter 22
Conclusion

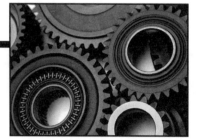

This book is one of a kind. It was written by an autistic medical professional who sees everything in health care facilities through autistic eyes. Not only do I have thirty-three years' experience in the medical profession, but I also have fifty-seven years of life with autism.

I can attest to the fact that it is a very daunting thing to go to a doctor's office just for a routine visit, or to somewhere more serious, like the Emergency Room. It is all stressful enough for the typical person but far beyond that, when you have ASD, which could lead those with ASD to avoid going to seek medical care to avoid all that goes with it. Additionally, knowing that health care providers don't understand autism or how to deal with it is also a factor among those who decide not to seek care. There are millions of individuals with ASD. They all deserve excellent health care, just like everyone else. Something has to be done to change the health care system as it stands right now. All health care providers must receive education about ASD and how to best care for these patients. Health care providers typically associate autism with children, because that has been the main focus. That paradigm is shifting as it becomes apparent that there are millions of adults with ASD.

Ever since getting diagnosed with autism seven years ago, I began conducting a little research of my own. In the operating room, there are frequently visiting medical students, surgery residents, nursing students, physical therapy students, physician's assistants, and others. I make a point to ask them what they know about autism and what they learned in their course of study about it. The resounding answer is nothing. Or, worse than that: they say things like "Oh, yes! We learned what age the onset is in children, but at least it goes away once they grow up." Or, "Autism is when a child has severe anger issues and has violent rages." My seven-year study concludes that this book is necessary. Every health care program must include this book in its curriculum. Diabetes, cardiovascular issues, and pulmonary diseases are all part of what's taught to health care providers. So too must be autism. It is a rapidly exploding condition that affects millions of children AND adults worldwide. Autism deserves the same degree of respect and seriousness. Just as diabetes affects the entire person, so does autism. We cannot wait any longer to get this as part of training across the nation and around the globe. Autism has no borders. It is in every country. Individuals with ASD need to be able to go for health care knowing that they will be understood and respected and cared for, just like everyone else.

When I set out to write this book, I didn't know what I'd find online. I was happy to see that a small but growing number of hospitals are realizing that it is necessary to provide specialty care for patients with ASD. However, based on what I found, they might be providing the dimly lit rooms, limiting staff that is caring for the ASD patient, and making quiet areas for them. However, very few are educating their staff about autism in addition to changing the environmental aspect. In fact, nowhere was it found that the staff members from the admissions desk through the final discharge were being educated about autism and how to best care for this unique population.

There was minimal data regarding health care for females with ASD. There are millions of female adults with ASD. This topic desperately needed to be addressed in this book. Every OB/GYN and anyone working in their offices needs to read Chapter 18. The focus of health care for those on the ASD spectrum always seems to be on males, but I wasn't about to let that happen here!

The chapters of this book were kept short and direct to enable the reader to grasp important concepts without going into too much detail. I tried to leave no stone unturned.

My goal is for my people, my fellow community with ASD, to feel confident to seek health care, to maintain good health, and to get issues treated. They should feel respected and taken seriously, not have to worry about contending with long waits in overcrowded waiting areas, not have doctors or nurses looking at them like they are crazy, and have health care providers treat them with dignity and patience. We didn't choose to be this way. As Temple Grandin's mother Eustacia Cutler says, we are "different … not less."

About the Author

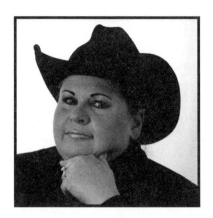

Anita was recently diagnosed with Asperger's Syndrome at age fifty. She graduated from Columbia University in New York City with a master of science degree in Nurse Anesthesia in 1988, and has been working ever since as an anesthetist, specializing in anesthesia for neurosurgery. Her special interests have earned her a flight in an F-15 fighter jet and jumping horses over 6 foot fences. An internationally recognized autism advocate and member of Autism Society of America's Panel of Autistic Advisors.

Anita is married to her husband Abraham, who is also autistic. They opened their wedding to the public to show that individuals with autism have a need for love, relationships and marriage just like everyone else. The event attracted international media attention including *People* and *Good Morning America*.

Anita is a Project Co-Lead on a $250,000 PCORI funded grant for Adults with Autism and other Stakeholders Engaging Together. This project aims to improve health and healthcare for autistic adults. She is a contributing author for numerous publications including the *Autism Asperger's Digest* and *The Mighty*. She is a blogger for the International Board of Credentialing and Continuing Education Standards. Anita's first book, *Asperger's Syndrome: When Life Hands You Lemons, Make Lemonade*, a memoir, was written immediately after she was diagnosed. She co-authored her second book, *Been There. Done That. Try This! The Aspie's Guide to Life on Earth*, with Dr. Tony Attwood and Craig Evans.

Anita is honored to have been a speaker at the United Nations Headquarters for World Autism Awareness Day 2017. She continues to work full time at her fast-paced, high stress job as Nurse Anesthetist while working tirelessly as an autism advocate.